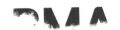

CHURCHILL'S POCKETBOOKS
ORTHOPAEDICS, TRAUMA AND RHEUMATOLOGY

WITHDRAWN
FROM LIBRARY

SECOND EDITION

CHURCHILL'S POCKETBOOKS

ORTHOPAEDICS, TRAUMA AND RHEUMATOLOGY

Andrew D. Duckworth MB ChB BSc MRCSEd MSc PhD

Specialty Registrar (StR) and Clinical Research Fellow, Edinburgh
Orthopaedic Trauma Unit, Royal Infirmary of Edinburgh, Edinburgh, UK

Daniel E. Porter MD FRCSEd(Orth)

Director of Department of Orthopaedic Surgery, First Affiliated Hospital of
Tsinghua University, Professor of Orthopaedic Surgery, Tsinghua
University Medical Centre, Beijing, China

Stuart H. Ralston MD FRCP FMedSci FRSE

Arthritis Research UK Professor of Rheumatology, Centre for Genomic
and Experimental Medicine, Institute of Genetics and Molecular Medicine,
Western General Hospital, Edinburgh, UK

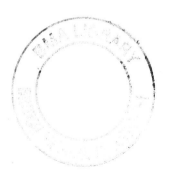

ELSEVIER

Edinburgh   London   New York   Oxford   Philadelphia
St Louis   Sydney   Toronto

ELSEVIER

First edition 2009
Second edition 2017

ISBN 978-0-7020-6318-3
International ISBN 978-0-7020-6317-6

Content Strategist: Laurence Hunter
Content Development Specialist: Helen Leng
Project Manager: Anne Collett
Designer: Miles Hitchen
Illustration Manager: Nichole Beard

ELSEVIER your source for books, journals and multimedia in the health sciences

www.elsevierhealth.com

Working together to grow libraries in developing countries

www.elsevier.com • www.bookaid.org

The publisher's policy is to use paper manufactured from sustainable forests

Printed in China
Last digit is the print number: 9 8 7 6 5 4 3 2 1

Contents

Preface

There continues to be a range of excellent undergraduate orthopaedic, rheumatology and trauma textbooks available to medical students and junior doctors alike. However, the authors have endeavoured to provide a fresh and concise pocket-sized single publication that covers all three topics at a level suitable for both trainees and junior doctors. In this second edition we have updated the content to reflect changes in surgical practice and advances in therapeutics, as well as the molecular understanding of genetic and inflammatory disorders.

The purpose of this text is not to replace the current recommended undergraduate texts within this specialty. It continues to have the ambition of providing an affordable pocket-sized adjunct to these texts, whilst also imparting much of the core knowledge needed as an undergraduate. As before, the text is aimed primarily at medical undergraduates for use during their placements in orthopaedics, A&E, rheumatology and general practice, as well as during their musculoskeletal anatomy course. However, with the new additions we hope it will also be a useful adjunct for junior doctors during any time spent in these specialties.

The handbook is designed to provide the essential points for each region with regards to anatomy, examination, investigations and management, whilst also providing succinct illustrations and figures where appropriate. In this second edition we hope that the reader will appreciate the updated layout and additions. The new 'overview' and 'hints and tips' boxes, as well as the addition of details on common procedures, aim to provide concise and important information not only to medical students revising for their exams, but also to junior doctors in their first years following graduation.

A.D.D.
D.E.P.
S.H.R.

Acknowledgements

The authors would again like to acknowledge those who provided invaluable advice with the first edition of the book. We would also like to thank Mr Tim White and Mr Paul Jenkins for their invaluable assistance with the procedure sections of the book, and Mr Sam Molyneux for his expertise with the trauma topics. We would also like to acknowledge Dr Catherine Collinson for her expert advice regarding the perioperative care section, and Mr Mark Hughes for his assistance with the head, neck and spine section.

We would like to thank our colleagues for their assistance with acquiring the new figures seen throughout the text, in particular Sam Mackenzie, as well as Mr Mark Gaston for his help with acquiring the figures for the paediatric section of the book.

As acknowledged in the first edition, we are forever indebted to Dr Mike Ford for allowing us to use the pictures from his text: *Introduction to Clinical Examination*.

Acronyms*

ABC	airway, breathing, circulation	**CVA**	cerebrovascular accident
ACE	angiotensin converting enzyme	**DDH**	developmental dysplasia of the hip
ACL	anterior cruciate ligament	**DEXA**	dual energy X-ray absorptiometry
ACPA	anti-citrullinated peptide antibodies	**DIC**	disseminated intravascular coagulation
ACS	acute compartment syndrome	**DIPJ**	distal interphalangeal joint
AIN	anterior interosseous nerve	**DMARDs**	disease-modifying antirheumatic drugs
ALP	alkaline phosphatase	**dsDNA**	double-stranded DNA
ANA	antinuclear antibody	**DVT**	deep vein thrombosis
ANCA	antineutrophil cytoplasmic antibody	**EPL**	extensor pollicis longus
AP	anteroposterior	**ESR**	erythrocyte sedimentation rate
APA	anti-phospholipid antibodies	**FBC**	full blood count
ARDS	acute respiratory distress syndrome	**FDP**	flexor digitorum profundus
ARF	acute renal failure	**FFD**	fixed flexion deformity
AS	ankylosing spondylitis	**FOOSH**	fall onto the palmar aspect of the hand; literally: fall onto outstretched hand
ASB	anatomical snuffbox		
AVN	avascular necrosis		
ATLS	advanced trauma life support	**GA**	general anaesthetic
BMD	bone mineral density	**GCA**	giant cell arteritis
CCP	cyclic citrullinated peptide	**GCS**	Glasgow Coma Scale
CK	creatine kinase	**HBV**	hepatitis B virus
CMCJ	carpometacarpal joint	**HLA**	human leukocyte antigen
COX	cyclo-oxygenase	**HO**	heterotopic ossification
CPDA	common palmar digital artery	**HRT**	hormone replacement therapy
CRP	C-reactive protein	**IBD**	inflammatory bowel disease
CRPS	chronic regional pain syndrome	**IBS**	irritable bowel syndrome
CT	computerized tomography	**Ig**	immunoglobulin
		IHD	ischaemic heart disease
CTD	connective tissue disease	**IPJ**	interphalangeal joint

*All acronyms used in this book are listed here unless the acronym is well known (e.g. CNS, ECG, MRI), has been used only once, or has been used only in figures or tables, in which case the acronym is defined in the figure legend or at the end of the table.

JIA	juvenile idiopathic arthritis
LA	local anaesthetic
LCL	lateral collateral ligament
LFTs	liver function tests
LMWH	low molecular weight heparin
LRTI	lower respiratory tract infection
MCL	medial collateral ligament
MCPJ	metacarpophalangeal joint
MHE	multiple hereditary exostoses
MI	myocardial infarction
MPA	microscopic polyangiitis
MRI	magnetic resonance imaging
MTPJ	metatarsophalangeal joint
MTX	methotrexate
MUA	manipulation under anaesthesia
NICE	National Institute for Health and Clinical Excellence
NSAIDs	non-steroidal anti-inflammatory drugs
OA	osteoarthritis
ORIF	open reduction and internal fixation
PA	posteroanterior
PAN	polyarteritis nodosa

PCL	posterior cruciate ligament
PE	pulmonary embolus
PET	positron emission tomography
PIPJ	proximal interphalangeal joint
PMR	polymyalgia rheumatica
POP	plaster of Paris
PPI	proton pump inhibitor
PsA	psoriatic arthritis
PTH	parathyroid hormone
PUD	peptic ulcer disease
RA	rheumatoid arthritis
RF	rheumatoid factor
ROM	range of motion
RTA	road traffic accident
SI	sacroiliac
SLE	systemic lupus erythematosus
SUFE	slipped upper femoral epiphysis
TFTs	thyroid function tests
TIA	transient ischaemic attack
TNF	tumour necrosis factor
UCL	ulnar collateral ligament
UEs	urea and electrolytes
USS	ultrasound scan
UTI	urinary tract infection
VTE	venous thromboembolism
WCC	white cell count
WHO	World Health Organisation

Chapter 1
Anatomy

CHAPTER OUTLINE

SHOULDER

Bones and Joints (Figure 1.1)

The pectoral girdle has three joints:

- The sternoclavicular joint (atypical saddle-type synovial fibrocartilage joint):
  - Is stabilized by the costoclavicular and sternoclavicular (anterior and posterior) ligaments
  - Is innervated by the medial supraclavicular nerve
  - Is supplied by the suprascapular and internal thoracic arteries
- The acromioclavicular joint (atypical plane-type synovial fibrocartilage joint):
  - Is stabilized by the acromioclavicular and coracoclavicular ligaments
  - Is innervated by the lateral pectoral, supraclavicular and axillary nerves
  - Is supplied by the suprascapular and internal thoracic arteries
- The shoulder (glenohumeral) joint:
  - Is a synovial ball-and-socket joint, with the head of the humerus articulating within the glenoid fossa of the scapula:
    - The shallow cavity is bordered by a lip of fibrocartilage known as the glenoid labrum that stabilizes the joint
    - The joint is encompassed within a flexible capsule, which runs from the glenoid labrum around to the anatomical neck
    - The capsule is reinforced by the rotator cuff tendons, the long head of biceps and the surrounding ligaments (glenohumeral, coracoacromial, coracohumeral, transverse humeral) but is still weak inferiorly
  - Is innervated by the axillary, suprascapular and lateral pectoral nerves
  - Is supplied by the suprascapular, and the anterior and posterior circumflex humeral arteries.

Muscles (Table 1.1 and Figure 1.2)

- Rotator cuff:
  - Infraspinatus: external/lateral rotation
  - Subscapularis: internal/medial rotation

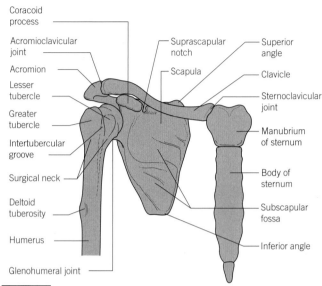

FIGURE 1.1

The pectoral girdle (anterior view).

- Supraspinatus: abduction
- Teres minor: external/lateral rotation
- Other muscles involved in the movement of the scapula are levator scapulae, rhomboid major and minor, pectoralis major and minor, trapezius, subclavius (clavicle) and serratus anterior
- Supraspinatus and deltoid are responsible for glenohumeral abduction:
  - Greater tuberosity impinges on glenoid labrum (~90°)
  - External rotation of arm provides further abduction to 90–120°
- Trapezius and serratus anterior provide abduction past ~120° by rotating the scapula, thus forcing the glenoid cavity to point superiorly.

Blood Supply

The axillary artery supplies the shoulder region:

- The origin is the subclavian artery, and it starts at the lateral border of the first rib surrounded by the axillary vein, lymph nodes and brachial plexus cords.
- Branches include the superior thoracic artery, thoracoacromial artery, lateral thoracic artery, subscapular artery and circumflex humeral arteries (anterior and posterior).
- It becomes the brachial artery at the inferior edge of teres major.

TABLE 1.1

THE MUSCLES, WITH THEIR INNERVATIONS, WHICH PROVIDE MOVEMENT AT THE SHOULDER JOINT*

Movement	Muscle	Origin	Insertion	Nerve
Abduction	Supraspinatus	Supraspinatus fossa of scapula	Greater tuberosity of humerus	Suprascapular
	Deltoid (m)	Acromion	Deltoid tuberosity of humerus	Axillary
Adduction	Latissimus dorsi	T6-T12, iliac crest, inferior ribs	Bicipital groove of humerus	Thoracodorsal
	Pectoralis major	Clavicle, sternum, upper six ribs	Bicipital groove of humerus	Pectoral nerves
	Teres major	Posterior–inferior aspect of scapula	Medial lip of humeral bicipital groove	Subscapular
	Coracobrachialis	Coracoid process of scapula	Medial aspect of humeral shaft	Musculocutaneous
	Subscapularis	Subscapular fossa	Lesser tubercle of humerus	Subscapular
Flexion	Deltoid (a)	Lateral third of clavicle	Deltoid tuberosity of humerus	Axillary
	Pectoralis major	Clavicle, sternum, upper six ribs	Bicipital groove of humerus	Pectoral nerves
	Coracobrachialis	Coracoid process of scapula	Medial aspect of humeral shaft	Musculocutaneous
Extension	Latissimus dorsi	T6-12, iliac crest, inferior ribs	Bicipital groove of humerus	Thoracodorsal
	Deltoid (p)	Spine of scapula	Deltoid tuberosity of humerus	Axillary
	Pectoralis major	Clavicle, sternum, upper six ribs	Bicipital groove of humerus	Pectoral nerves
Medial rotation	Latissimus dorsi	T6-T12, iliac crest, inferior ribs	Bicipital groove of humerus	Thoracodorsal
	Pectoralis major	Clavicle, sternum, upper six ribs	Bicipital groove of humerus	Pectoral nerves
	Teres major	Posterior–inferior aspect of scapula	Medial lip of humeral bicipital groove	Subscapular
	Deltoid (a)	Lateral third of clavicle	Deltoid tuberosity of humerus	Axillary
	Subscapularis	Subscapular fossa	Lesser tuberosity of humerus	Subscapular
Lateral rotation	Deltoid (p)	Spine of scapula	Deltoid tuberosity of humerus	Axillary
	Teres minor	Lateral border of scapula	Greater tuberosity of humerus	Axillary
	Infraspinatus	Infraspinous fossa of scapula	Greater tuberosity of humerus	Suprascapular

*Pectoralis major contributes to both shoulder flexion and extension, and is innervated by the lateral and medial pectoral nerves. It has two heads: clavicular (shoulder flexion) and sternocostal (shoulder extension). Coracobrachialis, an anterior compartment muscle of the arm, provides minor contributions to shoulder flexion and adduction.

a, anterior fibres of deltoid; m, middle fibres of deltoid; p, posterior fibres of deltoid.

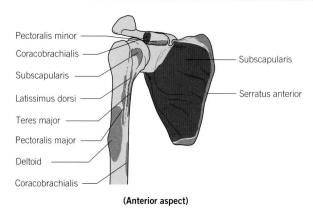

(Anterior aspect)

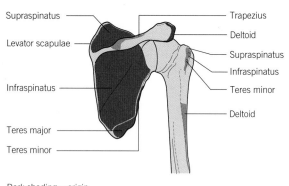

Dark shading = origin
Light shading = insertion

(Posterior aspect)

FIGURE 1.2

The muscles that contribute to movement at the shoulder joint.

Brachial Plexus (Figure 1.3)

- Brachial plexus arises from the ventral rami C5-T1 and the branches innervate the shoulder region as well as the rest of the upper limb:
  - Roots (C5-T1): scalenus anterior and medius
  - Trunks (superior C5-C6, middle C7, inferior C8-T1): posterior triangle of the neck
  - Divisions (anterior or posterior): posterior to the clavicle
  - Cords (lateral, posterior, medial): axilla

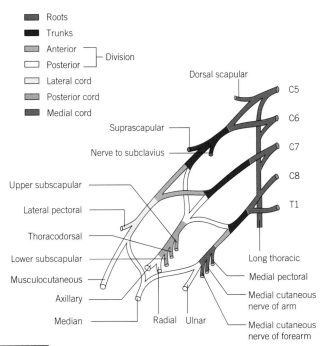

FIGURE 1.3

The brachial plexus.

- Axillary nerve:
  - Arises from the C5-C6 roots (posterior cord) of the brachial plexus
  - Runs deep to deltoid with the circumflex humeral arteries around the surgical neck of the humerus
  - Gives sensory cutaneous divisions to the lateral aspect of the upper arm, i.e. over the deltoid
  - Gives muscular innervations to the deltoid and teres minor.

 HINTS AND TIPS

SHOULDER

The anatomical neck of the humerus is located between the humeral head and the tubercles. The bicipital groove separates the tubercles, and the surgical neck marks the border between the proximal humerus and the humeral shaft. Hilton's law states that the nerve that innervates a joint often innervates the overlying

Continued

skin, as well as the muscles that move the joint. Traction injuries to the plexus can lead to characteristic findings. An upper plexus injury (C5-C6) is often secondary to a downward traction on the arm, resulting in an Erb–Duchenne palsy that gives a classic 'waiter's tip' position to the limb. An upward traction injury normally leads to a lower plexus injury (C8-T1) resulting in a Klumpke palsy giving a clawed hand. A lesion of T1 (e.g. Pancoast tumour, cervical rib) can result in Horner's syndrome with ptosis, miosis and anhidrosis.

ELBOW

Bones and Joints (Figure 1.4)

The elbow joint:

- Is a hinged synovial joint that comprises three articular points:
  - Medially, the humeral trochlea articulates with the trochlear notch of the ulna
  - Laterally, the proximal radial head articulates with the humeral capitellum
  - The proximal radioulnar joint
- Is encompassed within a flexible capsule, which is weaker anteriorly and posteriorly but is reinforced by the radial (laterally) and ulnar (medially) collateral ligaments
- Is innervated by the radial and musculocutaneous nerves, with small contributions from the median and ulnar nerves.

Muscles (Table 1.2 and Figure 1.5)

The arm has an anterior and a posterior compartment divided by septa (medial and lateral intermuscular septa) formed from the deep fascia:

- Anterior (flexor) compartment (biceps brachii, brachialis, coracobrachialis):
  - Is innervated by the musculocutaneous nerve, apart from brachialis which is also supplied by the radial nerve
  - Biceps brachii has two heads (long and short) and is the strongest muscle responsible for forearm supination
  - Coracobrachialis contributes to shoulder flexion and adduction
- Posterior (extensor) compartment (triceps):
  - Is innervated by the radial nerve
  - Triceps has three heads (long, medial, lateral).

Blood Supply

The brachial artery supplies both the anterior and posterior compartments of the arm:

- The origin is the axillary artery and it starts at the inferior edge of teres major
- It branches to give:
  - Profunda brachii that runs in the humeral spiral groove and supplies both compartments of the arm
  - Superior and inferior ulnar collateral arteries that supply the elbow joint

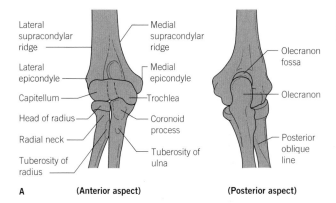

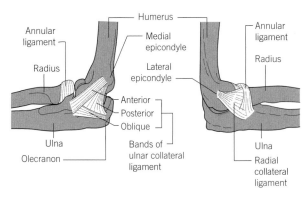

FIGURE 1.4

(**A**) The elbow joint. (**B**) The elbow joint is stabilized by surrounding collateral (lateral and medial complexes) and annular ligaments.

- It becomes the radial and ulnar arteries at the radial neck (early/high bifurcation possible).

Nerves

- The musculocutaneous nerve (Figure 1.6) innervates the anterior compartment of the arm:
  - It arises from the C5-C7 roots (lateral cord) of the brachial plexus
  - It pierces coracobrachialis and then passes obliquely between biceps brachii and brachialis
  - It terminates as the lateral cutaneous nerve of the forearm

---

TABLE 1.2

THE MUSCLES, WITH THEIR INNERVATIONS, WHICH PROVIDE MOVEMENT AT THE ELBOW JOINT*

Movement	Muscle	Origin	Insertion	Nerve
Elbow flexion	Biceps brachii			Musculocutaneous
	Long	Supraglenoid tuberosity	Radial tuberosity	
	Short	Coracoid process	Radial tuberosity	
	Brachialis	Anterior aspect of humerus	Ulnar coronoid process and tuberosity	Musculocutaneous, radial
	Pronator teres	Common flexor origin and coronoid process of ulnar	Lateral aspect of radius	Median
	Brachioradialis	Lateral supracondyle of humerus	Distal radius (styloid process)	Radial
Elbow extension	Triceps brachii			Radial
	Long	Infraglenoid tubercle of scapula	Olecranon process of ulna	
	Lateral	Superior to radial sulcus	Olecranon process of ulna	
	Medial	Inferior to radial sulcus	Olecranon process of ulna	
	Anconeus	Lateral epicondyle of humerus	Olecranon process and shaft of ulna	Radial

*Pronation and supination of the forearm does not occur exclusively at the elbow (see Table 1.5). Brachioradialis and the humeral head of pronator teres (an anterior compartment muscle of the forearm) both contribute to elbow flexion. Anconeus contributes to elbow extension.

- The radial nerve (Figure 1.7) innervates the posterior compartments of the arm and forearm:
  - It arises from the C5-T1 roots (posterior cord) of the brachial plexus
  - It traverses the lower triangular space (triangular interval) of the axilla, between the medial and long head of triceps, and enters the posterior compartment of the arm running posterior to the axillary artery:
    - Sensory cutaneous division to posterior aspect of the arm
  - It runs down the posteromedial aspect of the arm, then within the humeral spinal groove with the profunda brachii vessels, and emerges posterolaterally
  - It pierces the lateral septum just superior to the elbow joint to enter the anterior compartment, passing between brachialis and brachioradialis, running lateral to the biceps tendon and then anterior to the lateral epicondyle:
    - Sensory cutaneous divisions to the posterior and lateral aspects of the arm, as well as the posterior forearm

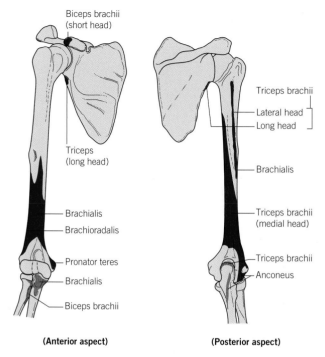

(Anterior aspect)   **(Posterior aspect)**

Dark shade = origin
Light shade = insertion

FIGURE 1.5

The muscles that contribute to movement at the elbow joint.

- It enters the forearm posterior to brachioradialis and branches to give the posterior interosseous nerve (deep motor) and the superficial radial nerve (sensory)
- The median nerve arises from the C6-T1 roots (lateral and medial cords) of the brachial plexus:
  - It enters the arm anterior to the distal third of the axillary artery
  - It crosses the brachial artery in the arm, moving from lateral to medial, both of which lie medial and superficial to the biceps tendon and brachialis respectively
  - It enters the forearm between the heads of pronator teres with no innervations in the arm
- The ulnar nerve arises from the C8-T1 roots (medial cord) of the brachial plexus:
  - It enters the arm medial to the axillary artery
  - It runs down the posteromedial aspect of the arm medially to the brachial artery and then pierces the medial septum

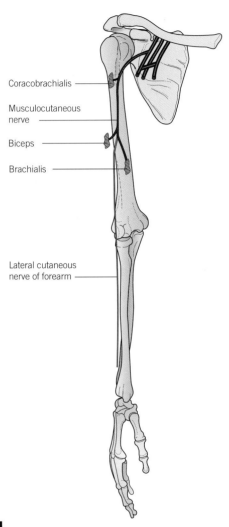

Coracobrachialis

Musculocutaneous nerve

Biceps

Brachialis

Lateral cutaneous nerve of forearm

FIGURE 1.6

The motor and sensory innervations from the musculocutaneous nerve.

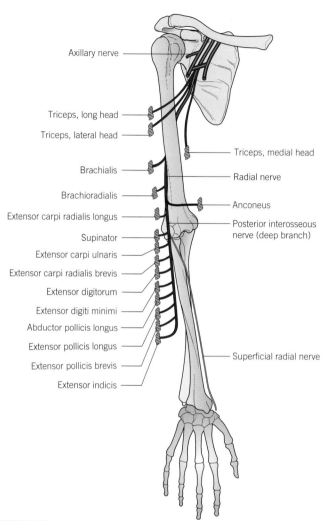

FIGURE 1.7
The motor and sensory innervations from the radial nerve.

- It passes posterior to the humeral medial epicondyle in the ulnar groove (funny bone) as it enters the forearm
- It enters the forearm between the heads of flexor carpi ulnaris with no innervations in the arm
- All four of these nerves (musculocutaneous, radial, median, ulnar) innervate the elbow joint and originate from the brachial plexus.

 HINTS AND TIPS

ELBOW

An injury to the radial nerve can occur in the axilla and would result in loss of elbow extension, wrist extension and MCPJ finger extension. However, a lesion in the spiral groove of the humerus, e.g. secondary to a humeral shaft fracture, results in preservation of elbow extension but with loss of wrist and MCPJ extension. The common flexor origin is found on the medial epicondyle of the humerus and the common extensor origin is found on the lateral epicondyle of the humerus. These are the sites involved in golfer's and tennis elbow respectively. The antecubital fossa is bordered by pronator teres (medially), brachioradialis (laterally) and an imaginary line between the epicondyles (superiorly). The mnemonic **TAN** aids in remembering the contents of the fossa (lateral to medial): biceps **t**endon, brachial **a**rtery and median **n**erve.

WRIST AND HAND

Bones and Joints (Figure 1.8)

The radioulnar joint is a pivot synovial joint and:

- Has a proximal and a distal joint, where pronation and supination occur
- Is innervated by:
  - Proximal: median, radial and musculocutaneous nerves
  - Distal: anterior and posterior interosseous nerves
- Is supplied by the anterior and posterior interosseous arteries.

The wrist joint:

- Is a condyloid synovial joint and comprises:
  - The proximal carpal bones (triquetrum, lunate, scaphoid) articulating with the distal radius and ulna, which are responsible predominantly for flexion/extension, abduction/adduction and circumduction of the wrist
  - The intercarpal joints which are plane synovial joints that are responsible predominantly for wrist abduction and flexion
  - The distal carpal bones (trapezium, trapezoid, capitate, hamate) with the metacarpals (CMCJs)
- Is reinforced by the intrinsic and extrinsic ligaments of the wrist
- Is innervated by the anterior interosseous (a branch of the median nerve) and the posterior interosseous (a branch of the radial nerve) nerves
- Is supplied by the palmar and dorsal carpal arterial arches.

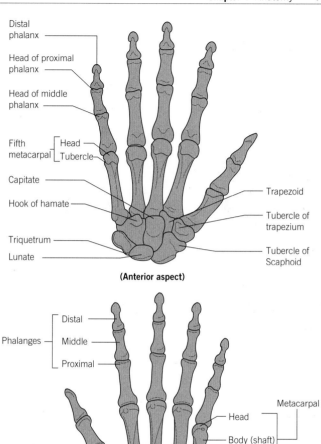

Distal phalanx

Head of proximal phalanx

Head of middle phalanx

Fifth metacarpal — Head / Tubercle

Capitate

Hook of hamate

Triquetrum

Lunate

Trapezoid

Tubercle of trapezium

Tubercle of Scaphoid

(Anterior aspect)

Phalanges — Distal / Middle / Proximal

Metacarpal — Head / Body (shaft) / Base

Trapezoid

Trapezium

Scaphoid

Lunate

Capitate

Hamate

Triquetrum

(Posterior aspect)

FIGURE 1.8

Bones of the right hand and wrist joint.

The hand joints:

- Include the carpometacarpal joints (CMCJs), MCPJs, PIPJs and DIPJs
- Are all synovial joints.

Muscles (Figure 1.9)

The forearm has an anterior and a posterior compartment divided by a robust interosseous membrane that connects the radius and ulna:

- Anterior (flexor) compartment:
  - Is innervated by the median (with its branch the anterior interosseous) and ulnar nerves
  - The flexor carpi ulnaris (ulnar and humeral), pronator teres (ulnar and humeral) and FDS (radial and humeroulnar) all have two heads
  - Is predominantly responsible for flexion of the wrist (Table 1.3), as well as flexion of the digital joints (Table 1.4)
  - The FDS and FDP are responsible for digital flexion (excluding the thumb) via attachment of long flexor tendons to the middle phalanx and terminal phalanx, respectively
  - Is also responsible for pronation of the forearm (Table 1.5) with pronator quadratus contributing to forearm pronation alone, whereas pronator teres also contributes to elbow flexion
- Posterior (extensor) compartment:
  - Is innervated by the radial nerve and its branch, the posterior interosseous nerve
  - Is predominantly responsible for extension of the wrist joint (Table 1.3), as well as extension of the digital joints. It also contributes to thumb extension and abduction (Table 1.4). The six extensor compartments of the wrist are (radial to ulnar):
    - Abductor pollicis longus and extensor pollicis brevis
    - Extensor carpi radialis longus and extensor carpi radialis brevis
    - Extensor pollicis longus
    - Extensor indicis and extensor digitorum communis
    - Extensor digiti minimi
    - Extensor carpi ulnaris
  - Is also responsible for supination of the forearm (Table 1.5) with supinator aiding the biceps brachii
  - Brachioradialis contributes to elbow flexion alone, whereas anconeus contributes to elbow extension alone.

The intrinsic muscles of the hand are often explained using three definable groups:

- Thenar eminence (abductor pollicis brevis, flexor pollicis brevis, opponens pollicis):
  - Is innervated by the recurrent branch of the median nerve
  - Is responsible for movements of the thumb (Table 1.4)
- Hypothenar eminence (abductor digiti minimi, flexor digiti minimi, opponens digiti minimi):

Text continued on p. 19

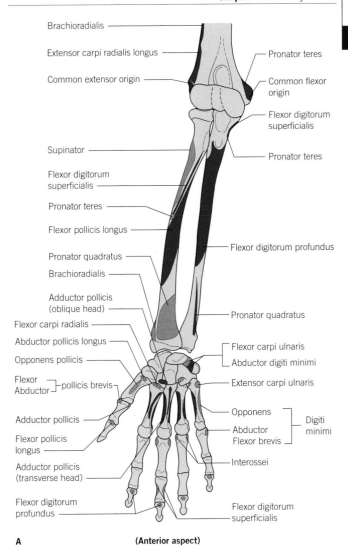

Brachioradialis

Extensor carpi radialis longus

Common extensor origin

Supinator

Flexor digitorum superficialis

Pronator teres

Flexor pollicis longus

Pronator quadratus

Brachioradialis

Adductor pollicis (oblique head)

Flexor carpi radialis

Abductor pollicis longus

Opponens pollicis

Flexor ┐pollicis brevis
Abductor ┘

Adductor pollicis

Flexor pollicis longus

Adductor pollicis (transverse head)

Flexor digitorum profundus

Pronator teres

Common flexor origin

Flexor digitorum superficialis

Pronator teres

Flexor digitorum profundus

Pronator quadratus

Flexor carpi ulnaris

Abductor digiti minimi

Extensor carpi ulnaris

Opponens ┐
Abductor ├ Digiti minimi
Flexor brevis ┘

Interossei

Flexor digitorum superficialis

A   **(Anterior aspect)**

FIGURE 1.9

The muscles that contribute to movement of the forearm and at the wrist and hand. (**A**) The volar/anterior compartment of the forearm. The long flexor tendons originate from muscles of the anterior compartment of the forearm and travel under the flexor retinaculum to insertion points on the metacarpals and phalanges via synovial flexor tendon sheaths.

Continued

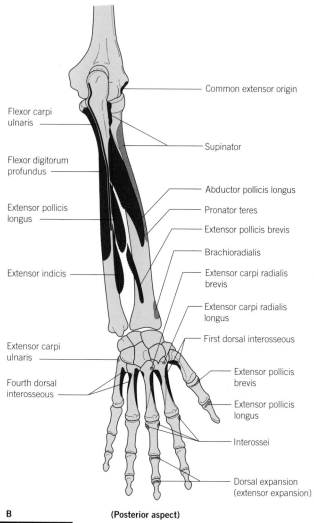

Common extensor origin

Flexor carpi
ulnaris

Supinator

Flexor digitorum
profundus

Abductor pollicis longus

Extensor pollicis
longus

Pronator teres

Extensor pollicis brevis

Brachioradialis

Extensor indicis

Extensor carpi radialis
brevis

Extensor carpi radialis
longus

First dorsal interosseous

Extensor carpi
ulnaris

Extensor pollicis
brevis

Fourth dorsal
interosseous

Extensor pollicis
longus

Interossei

Dorsal expansion
(extensor expansion)

B   **(Posterior aspect)**

FIGURE 1.9, cont'd

(**B**) The dorsal/posterior compartment of the forearm. The long extensor tendons
follow a similar path on the dorsal surface, again within synovial sheaths, and insert
into the middle and distal phalanges.

TABLE 1.3

THE MUSCLES, WITH THEIR INNERVATIONS, WHICH PROVIDE MOVEMENT AT THE WRIST JOINT*

Movement	Muscle	Origin	Insertion	Nerve
Wrist abduction	Extensor carpi radialis longus (PS)	Lateral supracondyle of humerus	Second metacarpal base	Radial
	Extensor carpi radialis brevis (PS)	Common extensor origin	Third metacarpal base	Posterior interosseous
	Flexor carpi radialis (AS)	Common flexor origin	Second metacarpal base	Median
Wrist adduction	Flexor carpi ulnaris (AS)			Ulnar
	Humeral head	Common flexor origin	Pisiform/fifth metacarpal	
	Ulnar head	Olecranon and posterior ulnar	Pisiform/fifth metacarpal	
	Extensor carpi ulnaris (PS)	Common extensor origin	Fifth metacarpal base	Posterior interosseous
Wrist flexion	Flexor carpi ulnaris (AS)	See above	See above	Ulnar
	Flexor carpi radialis (AS)	Common flexor origin	Second metacarpal base	Median
	Palmaris longus (AS)	Common flexor origin	Palmar aponeurosis	Median
	Flexor digitorum superficialis (AS)	Common flexor origin, coronoid process, radius	Four middle phalanges	Median
	Flexor digitorum profundus (AD)	Ulnar and interosseous membrane	Four distal phalanges	Ulnar/anterior interosseous
Wrist extension	Extensor carpi radialis longus (PS)	Lateral supracondyle of humerus	Second metacarpal base	Radial
	Extensor carpi radialis brevis (PS)	Common extensor origin	Third metacarpal base	Posterior interosseous
	Extensor carpi ulnaris (PS)	Common extensor origin	Fifth metacarpal base	Posterior interosseous
	Extensor digitorum (PS)	Common extensor origin	Extensor expansions of four ulnar middle/distal phalanges	Posterior interosseous

*Flexor digitorum profundus is supplied by the ulnar nerve medially (ring and little fingers) and the anterior interosseous nerve laterally (index and middle fingers).

A, anterior compartment of forearm; D, deep; P, posterior compartment of forearm; S, superficial.

TABLE 1.4

THE MUSCLES, WITH THEIR INNERVATIONS, WHICH PROVIDE MOVEMENT OF THE THUMB AND FINGERS*

Movement	Muscle	Origin	Insertion	Nerve
Thumb abduction	Abductor pollicis longus (PD)	Ulnar and radius	First MC base	Posterior interosseous
	Abductor pollicis brevis (TS)	Scaphoid, trapezium, FR	Thumb proximal phalanx	Recurrent branch median
Thumb adduction	Adductor pollicis (I)	Capitate, trapezoid, second/third MC	Thumb proximal phalanx	Deep branch ulnar
Thumb flexion	Flexor pollicis longus (AD)	Radius and interosseous membrane	Thumb distal phalanx	Anterior interosseous
	Flexor pollicis brevis (TS)	Trapezium, FR	Thumb proximal phalanx	Recurrent branch median
Thumb extension	Extensor pollicis brevis (PD)	Radius and interosseous membrane	Thumb proximal phalanx	Posterior interosseous
	Extensor pollicis longus (PD)	Ulnar and interosseous membrane	Thumb distal phalanx	Posterior interosseous
Fifth digit abduction	Abductor digiti minimi (HS)	Pisiform, FR	Fifth digit proximal phalanx	Deep branch ulnar
Fifth digit flexion	Flexor digiti minimi (HS)	Hook of hamate, FR	Fifth digit proximal phalanx	Deep branch ulnar
Fifth digit extension	Extensor digiti minimi (PS)	Common extensor origin	Extensor expansion of 5th digit	Posterior interosseous
Digital abduction	Dorsal interossei (I)	Metacarpals	Base proximal phalanges	Deep branch ulnar
Digital adduction	Palmar interossei (I)	Metacarpals	Base proximal phalanges	Deep branch ulnar
Digital flexion	FDS (AS)	See Table 1.3	See Table 1.3	Median
	FDP (AD)	See Table 1.3	See Table 1.3	Ulnar/anterior interosseous
Digital extension	Extensor digitorum (PS)	Common extensor origin	Extensor expansions of 4 ulnar middle/distal phalanges	Posterior interosseous

*Extensor indicis, a posterior compartment muscle of the forearm, contributes to second digit extension alone. Opponens pollicis and opponens digiti minimi medially rotate the thumb and fifth digit, respectively, creating opposition, thus producing a grip that is also aided by palmaris brevis.

A, anterior compartment of forearm; D, deep; FR, flexor retinaculum; H, hypothenar eminence; I, intrinsic muscle of hand; MC, metacarpal; P, posterior compartment of forearm; S, superficial; T, thenar eminence.

TABLE 1.5

THE MUSCLES, WITH THEIR INNERVATIONS, WHICH PROVIDE MOVEMENT AT THE RADIOULNAR JOINT**

Movement	Muscle	Origin	Insertion	Nerve
Pronation	Pronator teres (AS)			Median
	Humeral head	Common flexor origin	Lateral aspect of radius	
	Ulnar head	Coronoid process of ulna	Lateral aspect of radius	
	Pronator quadratus (AD)	Anteromedial aspect of ulna	Anterolateral aspect of radius	Anterior interosseous
Supination	Supinator (PS)	Common extensor origin, elbow ligaments, crest of ulna	Radial neck and shaft	Posterior interosseous
	Biceps brachii	See Table 1.2	See Table 1.2	See Table 1.2

*Biceps brachii, an anterior compartment muscle of the arm, contributes to supination. Anconeus, a posterior compartment muscle of the forearm, contributes to movement of the ulna during pronation.

A, anterior compartment of forearm; D, deep; P, posterior compartment of forearm; S, superficial.

- Is innervated by the deep branch of the ulnar nerve
- Is responsible for movements of the little finger (Table 1.4)
- Other intrinsic muscles (palmar interossei, dorsal interossei, lumbricals, adductor pollicis):
  - Are innervated by the deep branch of the ulnar nerve and the median nerve
  - Are responsible for abduction and adduction of the digits, as well as MCPJ flexion/IPJ extension (Table 1.4)
  - The adductor pollicis is responsible for thumb adduction alone.

Blood Supply (Figure 1.10)

The radial and ulnar arteries supply both the anterior and posterior compartments of the forearm and the hand:

- Ulnar artery:
  - Runs inferior to the common flexor origin and then between FDP and flexor carpi ulnaris in the forearm
  - Runs lateral to the ulnar nerve in the distal forearm and wrist
  - Gives rise early to the common interosseous artery, which divides to produce the anterior interosseous artery and the posterior interosseous artery – these two vessels re-join to supply the dorsum of the hand
  - Enters the hand superficial to the flexor retinaculum to give rise to the superficial palmar arch, from where it supplies the digits via the common palmar digital arteries (CPDAs)
- Radial artery:
  - Runs between flexor carpi radialis and brachioradialis in the forearm
  - Enters the hand via the anatomical snuffbox (deep to abductor pollicis longus and extensor pollicis brevis tendons) to give rise to the deep

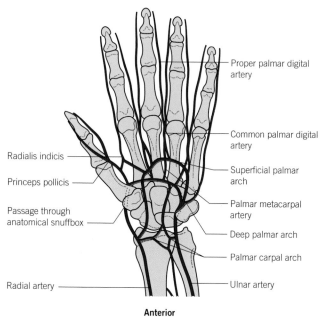

Proper palmar digital artery

Common palmar digital artery

Superficial palmar arch

Palmar metacarpal artery

Deep palmar arch

Palmar carpal arch

Ulnar artery

Radialis indicis

Princeps pollicis

Passage through anatomical snuffbox

Radial artery

Anterior

FIGURE 1.10

The blood supply of the wrist joint and hand.

palmar arch, from where it supplies the digits via branches that anastomose with the CPDAs.

Nerves

- Median nerve (Figure 1.11) enters the forearm between the heads of pronator teres and descends the forearm between FDP and FDS, innervating some of the anterior compartment:
  - An early branch is the anterior interosseous nerve, which innervates some of the muscles in the anterior compartment of the forearm
  - The nerve is superficial and in the midline at the wrist, entering the hand via the carpal tunnel (inferior to the flexor retinaculum and superolaterally to the tendons of FDS/FDP) and innervates the muscles of the thenar eminence as well as the first and second (radial) lumbricals. Branches at the wrist include:
  - The palmar branch (which supplies the skin over the thenar eminence), which passes superior to the flexor retinaculum, just superior to the wrist
  - The sensory cutaneous divisions to the central and radial aspect of the palm, and the radial 3.5 digits (Figure 1.12)

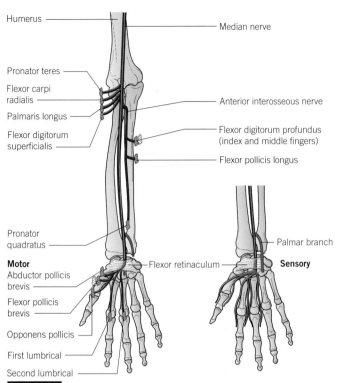

FIGURE 1.11

The motor and sensory innervations from the median nerve.

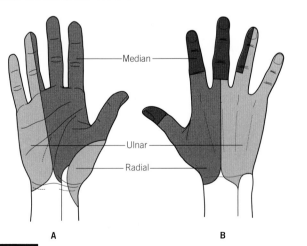

FIGURE 1.12

Sensory innervation of the hand: (**A**) anterior; (**B**) posterior.

- Ulnar nerve (Figure 1.13) enters the forearm between the heads of flexor carpi ulnaris, innervating some of the muscles in the anterior compartment:
  - In the forearm it runs between FDP and flexor carpi ulnaris, medial to the ulnar artery:
    - The palmar and dorsal (prior to Guyon's canal) branches that provide cutaneous innervation to the medial palm and ulnar 1.5 digits (Figure 1.12)
  - It enters the hand via Guyon's canal (with the ulnar artery) superficial to the flexor retinaculum and innervates the remaining intrinsic muscles of the hand
- Radial nerve (Figure 1.7) enters the forearm posterior to brachioradialis, innervating the posterior compartment of the forearm. It divides into the:
  - Posterior interosseous nerve (deep motor), which passes between the two heads of supinator and innervates the muscles in the posterior compartment of the forearm, as well as the wrist joint
  - Superficial radial nerve that travels down the forearm posterior to brachioradialis and provides sensory cutaneous divisions to the lateral dorsum of the hand (Figure 1.12).

 HINTS AND TIPS

WRIST AND HAND

The carpal tunnel contains the median nerve, the four tendons each of FDP and FDS as well as flexor pollicis longus. FCR is not within the tunnel and is found anterolateral to the flexor retinaculum. The mnemonic **PAd DAb** is related to the function of the interossei. The **p**almar interossei **ad**duct the finger whilst the **d**orsal interossei **ab**duct the fingers. The palmar aponeurosis is a thick sheet that connects the thenar and hypothenar muscles across the hand. Thickening and contracture of the aponeurosis as it extends into the digits leads to the characteristic deformity seen in Dupuytren's contracture (see Chapter 6).

HIP AND KNEE

Bones and Joints

The hip joint (Figure 1.14):

- Is a highly stable synovial ball-and-socket joint that is covered with hyaline cartilage and comprises the femoral head articulating within the acetabulum of the pelvis, which is bordered by a lip of fibrocartilage, known as the acetabular labrum, that stabilizes the joint:
  - Ligamentum teres passes from the femoral head fovea to the margins of the acetabular notch
- Is encompassed within a flexible capsule, which is reinforced and stabilized by the surrounding ligaments (iliofemoral, pubofemoral, ischiofemoral)
- Is innervated by the sciatic, femoral and obturator nerves
- Is supplied by the obturator, medial and lateral circumflex femoral and the superior and inferior gluteal arteries (the latter four forming the trochanteric anastomosis).

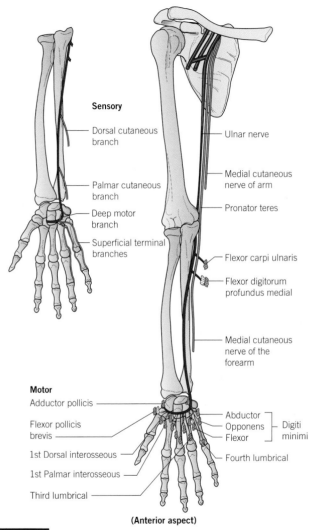

Sensory

- Dorsal cutaneous branch
- Palmar cutaneous branch
- Deep motor branch
- Superficial terminal branches

- Ulnar nerve
- Medial cutaneous nerve of arm
- Pronator teres
- Flexor carpi ulnaris
- Flexor digitorum profundus medial
- Medial cutaneous nerve of the forearm

Motor

- Adductor pollicis
- Flexor pollicis brevis
- 1st Dorsal interosseous
- 1st Palmar interosseous
- Third lumbrical

- Abductor ⎤
- Opponens ⎬ Digiti minimi
- Flexor ⎦
- Fourth lumbrical

(Anterior aspect)

FIGURE 1.13

The motor and sensory innervations from the ulnar nerve.

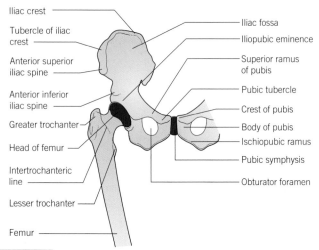

Iliac crest

Tubercle of iliac crest

Anterior superior iliac spine

Anterior inferior iliac spine

Greater trochanter

Head of femur

Intertrochanteric line

Lesser trochanter

Femur

Iliac fossa

Iliopubic eminence

Superior ramus of pubis

Pubic tubercle

Crest of pubis

Body of pubis

Ischiopubic ramus

Pubic symphysis

Obturator foramen

FIGURE 1.14

The hip joint is a stable and highly mobile ball-and-socket synovial joint.

The knee joint (Figure 1.15):

- Is a synovial hinge joint that is covered with hyaline cartilage and comprises:
  - The femoral condyles articulating with the proximal tibial condyles with medial and lateral compartments
  - The patella articulating with femur (patellofemoral joint)
- Is encompassed within a flexible incomplete capsule, which is reinforced and stabilized by tendons (e.g. from the quadriceps muscles) and the surrounding ligaments (patella, LCL, MCL, ACL, PCL, oblique, arcuate popliteal), as well as the patella itself:
  - The weaker ACL arises from the posteromedial aspect of the lateral femoral condyle, runs obliquely and inserts into the anterior intercondylar area of the tibia
  - The PCL arises from the anterolateral aspect of the medial femoral condyle and inserts into the posterior intercondylar area of the tibia
- Has menisci, which are crescent-shaped mobile wedges that aid load bearing
  - They are found attached to the superior surface of the tibia and surrounding ligaments:
  - The medial meniscus is larger than the lateral
- Is innervated by the femoral, sciatic (tibial and common peroneal) and obturator nerves
- Is supplied by the branches from the genicular anastomoses (e.g. from the popliteal artery).

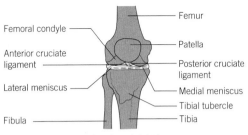

Femur

Femoral condyle

Patella

Anterior cruciate ligament

Posterior cruciate ligament

Lateral meniscus

Medial meniscus

Tibial tubercle

Fibula

Tibia

Anterior view of right knee

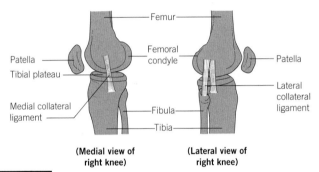

Femur

Femoral condyle

Patella

Tibial plateau

Patella

Lateral collateral ligament

Medial collateral ligament

Fibula

Tibia

(Medial view of right knee)

(Lateral view of right knee)

FIGURE 1.15

Bones and ligaments of the knee joint.

Muscles (Figure 1.16)

The superior and inferior gluteal nerves innervate the gluteal muscles. Their prominent role is in hip abduction, along with medial and lateral rotation. The anterior fibres of gluteus medius provide a minor contribution to external rotation of the hip, whilst the posterior fibres provide a minor contribution to lateral rotation. Gluteus maximus contributes to hip extension.

The thigh has three compartments – anterior, adductor and posterior – divided and encompassed by intermuscular septa and fascia lata:

- Anterior compartment (quadriceps femoris, iliacus, psoas major, sartorius, pectineus):
  - Is innervated by the femoral nerve, apart from psoas major that is innervated by the lumbar plexus, and pectineus that is partially innervated by the obturator nerve
  - Is responsible for movements at the hip and knee joints (Tables 1.6 and 1.7)

Text continued on p. 30

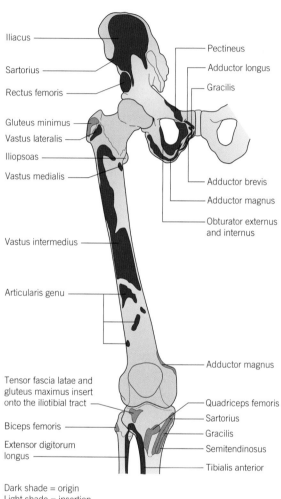

Iliacus

Sartorius

Rectus femoris

Gluteus minimus

Vastus lateralis

Iliopsoas

Vastus medialis

Vastus intermedius

Articularis genu

Tensor fascia latae and gluteus maximus insert onto the iliotibial tract

Biceps femoris

Extensor digitorum longus

Pectineus

Adductor longus

Gracilis

Adductor brevis

Adductor magnus

Obturator externus and internus

Adductor magnus

Quadriceps femoris

Sartorius

Gracilis

Semitendinosus

Tibialis anterior

Dark shade = origin
Light shade = insertion

A   (Anterior aspect)

FIGURE 1.16

The (**A**) anterior and (**B**) posterior muscles that contribute to movement of the lower limb. The femoral triangle contains the femoral nerve, artery, vein and canal (the latter three encompassed within the femoral sheath), as well as the deep inguinal lymph nodes. The borders of the triangle are the inguinal ligament (superiorly), the medial border of adductor longus muscle (medially) and the medial border of the sartorius muscle (laterally).

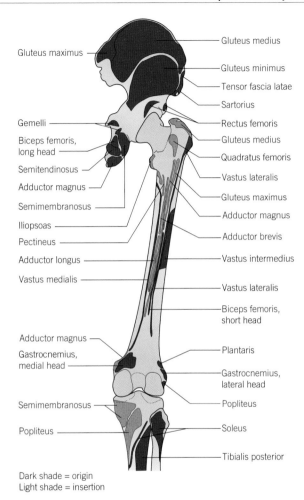

Gluteus medius

Gluteus maximus

Gluteus minimus

Tensor fascia latae

Sartorius

Rectus femoris

Gemelli

Gluteus medius

Biceps femoris, long head

Quadratus femoris

Semitendinosus

Vastus lateralis

Adductor magnus

Gluteus maximus

Semimembranosus

Adductor magnus

Iliopsoas

Adductor brevis

Pectineus

Adductor longus

Vastus intermedius

Vastus medialis

Vastus lateralis

Biceps femoris, short head

Adductor magnus

Plantaris

Gastrocnemius, medial head

Gastrocnemius, lateral head

Semimembranosus

Popliteus

Popliteus

Soleus

Tibialis posterior

Dark shade = origin
Light shade = insertion

B   **(Posterior aspect)**

FIGURE 1.16, cont'd

The adductor (Hunter) canal runs from the femoral triangle apex to the adductor hiatus. It contains the femoral artery and vein, along with the saphenous nerve. The borders are sartorius (anteromedially), vastus medialis (anterolaterally) and adductor longus and magnus (posteriorly/floor). The popliteal fossa is located in the posterior aspect of the knee and contains the popliteal vessels, branches of the sciatic nerve, as well as lymph nodes and bursa. The borders of the fossa are semimembranosus and semitendinosus (superomedially), biceps femoris (superolaterally), with the lateral and medial heads of gastrocnemius (inferiorly).

TABLE 1.6

THE MUSCLES, WITH THEIR INNERVATIONS, WHICH PROVIDE MOVEMENT AT THE HIP JOINT

Movement	Muscle	Origin	Insertion	Nerve
Abduction	Gluteus medius (G)	Ilium	Greater trochanter of femur	Superior gluteal
	Gluteus minimus (G)	Ilium	Greater trochanter of femur	Superior gluteal
	Sup. and inf. gemellus (G)	Ischial spine and tuberosity	Greater trochanter of femur	L5-S1 (sacral plexus)
Adduction	Pectineus (A)	Superior pubic ramus	Lesser trochanter of femur	Femoral
	Adductor brevis (M)	Inferior pubic ramus	Posterior aspect of femur	Obturator
	Adductor longus (M)	Body of pubis	Posterior aspect of femur	Obturator
	Adductor magnus (M)	Ischiopubic ramus	Posterior aspect of femur	Obturator, sciatic
	Gracilis (M)	Ischiopubic ramus	Superior/medial aspect of tibia	Obturator
Medial rotation	Gluteus minimus (G)	Ilium	Greater trochanter of femur	Superior gluteal
	Tensor fascia lata (G)	Iliac crest and ASIS	Iliotibial tract	Superior gluteal
Lateral rotation	Quadratus femoris (G)	Ischial tuberosity	Intertrochanteric crest of femur	L5-S1 (sacral plexus)
	Obturator internus (G)	Obturator membrane	Greater trochanter of femur	L5-S1 (sacral plexus)
	Piriformis (G)	Anterior aspect of sacrum	Greater trochanter of femur	Piriformis
	Sartorius (A)	Anterior superior iliac spine	Superior/medial aspect of tibia	Femoral
	Obturator externus (M)	Obturator membrane	Greater trochanter of femur	Obturator
	Sup. and inf. gemellus (G)	Ischial spine and tuberosity	Greater trochanter of femur	L5-S1 (sacral plexus)
Flexion	Sartorius (A)	Anterior superior iliac spine	Tibia	Femoral
	Psoas major (A)	Spine (T12-5)	Lesser trochanter of femur	L1-3 (lumbar plexus)
	Iliacus (A)	Iliac crest and fossa	Lesser trochanter of femur	Femoral
	Pectineus (A)	Superior pubic ramus	Femoral shaft	Femoral
	Rectus femoris (A)	AIIS (straight head)	Patellar tendon onto tibia	Femoral
		Acetabular rim (reflected head)		

TABLE 1.6

THE MUSCLES, WITH THEIR INNERVATIONS, WHICH PROVIDE MOVEMENT AT THE HIP JOINT—cont'd

Movement	Muscle	Origin	Insertion	Nerve
Extension	Gluteus maximus (G)	Ilium, coccyx, sacrum, sacrotuberous ligament	Gluteal tuberosity of the femur, iliotibial tract	Inferior gluteal
	Biceps femoris (P)	Ischial tuberosity and posterior aspect of femur	Fibula head	Tibial, common peroneal
	Semimembranosus (P)	Ischial tuberosity	Tibia (medial condyle)	Tibial
	Semitendinosus (P)	Ischial tuberosity	Tibia (superomedial aspect)	Tibial

Those muscles attaching to the posterior aspect of the femur will predominantly do so via the linea aspera of the femur.
A, anterior compartment of thigh; G, gluteal region; M, medial compartment of thigh; P, posterior compartment of thigh; AIIS, anterior inferior iliac spine; ASIS, anterior superior iliac spine.

TABLE 1.7

THE MUSCLES, WITH THEIR INNERVATIONS, WHICH PROVIDE MOVEMENT AT THE KNEE JOINT*

Movement	Muscle	Origin	Insertion	Nerve
Flexion	Sartorius (A)	ASIS	Superior/medial aspect of tibia	Femoral
	Gracilis (M)	Ischiopubic ramus	Superior/medial aspect of tibia	Obturator
	Biceps femoris (P)	Ischial tuberosity and posterior aspect of femur	Fibula head	Tibial, common peroneal
	Semimembranosus (P)	Ischial tuberosity	Tibia (medial condyle)	Tibial
	Semitendinosus (P)	Ischial tuberosity	Tibia (superomedial aspect)	Tibial
Extension	Rectus femoris (A)	AIIS (straight head) Acetabular rim (reflected head)	Patellar tendon onto tibia	Femoral
	Vastus medialis (A)	Upper aspect of femur	Patellar tendon onto tibia	Femoral
	Vastus lateralis (A)	Upper aspect of femur	Patellar tendon onto tibia	Femoral
	Vastus intermedius (A)	Body of femur	Patellar tendon onto tibia	Femoral

*The quadriceps is a group of muscles including vastus medialis, vastus lateralis, vastus intermedius and rectus femoris. Gastrocnemius and plantaris, posterior compartment muscles of the leg, provide minor contributions to knee flexion. The posterior compartment muscles are responsible for lateral and medial rotation of the knee joint when it is in flexion. Locking and unlocking of the knee are controlled by the surrounding ligaments and the popliteus muscle, respectively.
A, anterior compartment of thigh; M, medial compartment of thigh; P, posterior compartment of thigh; AIIS, anterior inferior iliac spine; ASIS, anterior superior iliac spine.

- Medial (adductor) compartment (adductor longus, brevis and magnus, obturator externus, gracilis):
  - Is innervated by the obturator nerve, apart from adductor magnus that is also innervated by the sciatic nerve (tibial division)
  - Is predominantly responsible for hip adduction (Tables 1.6 and 1.7)
  - The horizontal fibres of adductor magnus provide a minor contribution to hip flexion, with the vertical fibres providing a minor contribution to hip extension
  - Adductor longus and brevis provide minor contributions to hip flexion
- Posterior compartment (biceps femoris, semimembranosus, semitendinosus):
  - Is innervated by the common peroneal and tibial nerves (sciatic nerve)
  - Is responsible for hip extension, as well as knee flexion and rotation (Tables 1.6 and 1.7)
  - Biceps femoris has two heads (long and short), with the long providing a minor contribution to hip extension.

Blood Supply

- Superior (lies above the piriformis as it passes through the foramen) and inferior gluteal arteries originate from the internal iliac artery and supply the gluteal muscles, as well as the hip joint. The internal pudendal artery also supplies some muscles of the gluteal region. All pass through the greater sciatic foramen
- Obturator artery originates from the internal iliac artery and supplies predominantly the adductor compartment of the thigh as well as the hip joint
- Common femoral artery supplies the anterior compartment of the thigh:
  - The origin is the external iliac artery and it starts at the inferior edge of the inguinal ligament
  - It divides into the superficial and deep femoral arteries. It is the deep femoral artery (with the vein, susceptible to injury in femoral shaft fractures) that supplies the posterior compartment of the thigh, and itself gives rise to the perforators and the medial and lateral circumflex femoral arteries
  - It becomes the popliteal artery at the adductor magnus hiatus
- Cruciate anastomosis (first perforator of the deep femoral, inferior gluteal, medial and lateral circumflex femoral arteries) supplies the posterior aspect of the femur and is a collateral blood supply if the femoral artery becomes compromised
- Popliteal artery:
  - Gives rise to the superior, middle and inferior genicular artery branches, which supply the knee joint; it also gives rise to the sural arteries that supply some muscles of the leg
  - It becomes the anterior and posterior tibial arteries at the inferior edge of the popliteus muscle.

Nerves (Figure 1.17)

- Lumbar and sacral plexuses innervate the lower limb:
  - Branches of the lumbar plexus (L1-L4) include the femoral, obturator, genitofemoral and ilioinguinal nerves, along with the lateral cutaneous nerve of the thigh:
    - Obturator nerve (L2-L4) enters through the obturator foramen innervating the adductor compartment of the thigh, with sensory cutaneous divisions of the medial aspect of the thigh
    - Femoral nerve (L2-L4) traverses through psoas major and enters deep to the inguinal ligament innervating the anterior compartment of the thigh. Branches include the saphenous nerve and sensory cutaneous divisions to the anterior and medial aspects of the thigh

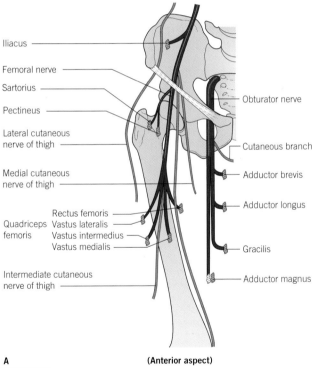

Iliacus

Femoral nerve

Sartorius

Pectineus

Lateral cutaneous nerve of thigh

Medial cutaneous nerve of thigh

Quadriceps femoris — Rectus femoris / Vastus lateralis / Vastus intermedius / Vastus medialis

Intermediate cutaneous nerve of thigh

Obturator nerve

Cutaneous branch

Adductor brevis

Adductor longus

Gracilis

Adductor magnus

A   **(Anterior aspect)**

FIGURE 1.17

The (**A**) anterior and (**B**) posterior motor and sensory innervations of the hip and knee region. The greater and lesser sciatic foramens are formed through the sacrospinous and sacrotuberous ligaments transecting the sciatic notches. In the greater sciatic foramen, the superior gluteal vessels and nerve pass superior to piriformis.

Continued

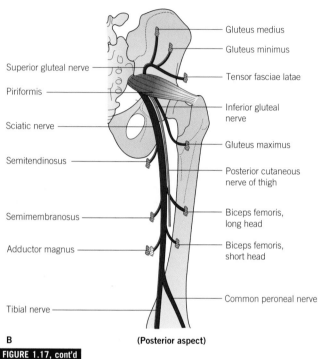

Gluteus medius

Gluteus minimus

Superior gluteal nerve

Tensor fasciae latae

Piriformis

Inferior gluteal nerve

Sciatic nerve

Gluteus maximus

Semitendinosus

Posterior cutaneous nerve of thigh

Semimembranosus

Biceps femoris, long head

Adductor magnus

Biceps femoris, short head

Common peroneal nerve

Tibial nerve

B   **(Posterior aspect)**

FIGURE 1.17, cont'd

- Branches of the sacral plexus (L4-L5 and S1-S4) include the superior and inferior gluteal, sciatic and pudendal nerves, along with the posterior cutaneous nerve of the thigh:
  - Superior gluteal nerve (L4-S1) exits the pelvis through the greater sciatic foramen (superior to piriformis), adjacent to the superior gluteal artery and vein. It passes between gluteus medius and minimus and ~4–5 cm above the greater trochanter, and provides innervation to gluteus medius/minimus and tensor fascia lata
  - Inferior gluteal nerve (L5-S2) exits the pelvis through the greater sciatic foramen (inferior to piriformis) and provides innervation to gluteus maximus
  - Sciatic nerve (L4-L5 and S1-S3) exits the pelvis through the greater sciatic foramen (inferior to piriformis), emerges deep to gluteus maximus and innervates the posterior compartment of the thigh (travelling between the hamstrings and adductor magnus) with two divisions that usually occur just superior to the knee joint – the common peroneal and tibial nerves. There are sensory innervations to the gluteal region and the posterior aspect of the thigh.

HINTS AND TIPS

HIP AND KNEE

The lateral and posterior approaches to the hip are commonly used for hip replacement surgery. The lateral approach involves splitting the fibres of gluteus medius and excessive splitting can lead to damage of the superior gluteal nerve. As a consequence there will be paralysis of the abductor muscles and clinically a Trendelenburg gait. The sciatic nerve is at risk during the posterior approach. The structures within the femoral triangle (from lateral to medial) are the femoral nerve, femoral artery, femoral vein and the femoral canal (mnemonic: **NAVY** = **n**erve, **a**rtery, **v**ein, **Y**-fronts). In the knee, due to the intimate relationship between the menisci and ligaments, damage to the ligaments can lead to an associated meniscal tear. The popliteal artery is the deepest structure of the popliteal fossa and is susceptible to damage following complex fractures around the knee or a knee dislocation.

ANKLE AND FOOT

Bones and Joints

The tibiofibular joint:

- Has proximal (superior) and distal (inferior) joints. The inferior joint is stabilized by the surrounding ligaments (anterior tibiofibular and posterior tibiofibular)
- Is innervated by:
  - Proximal: common peroneal nerve
  - Distal: deep peroneal, saphenous and tibial nerves
- Is supplied by:
  - Proximal: anterior tibial and inferior lateral genicular arteries
  - Distal: anterior and posterior tibial arteries.

The ankle joint (Figure 1.18):

- Is a stable hinged synovial joint covered with cartilage and comprises:
  - The distal inferior surfaces of the fibula and tibia (the lateral and medial malleoli, respectively) articulating with the superior surface body of the talus bone
- Is encompassed within a loose capsule, which is reinforced and stabilized by the surrounding ligaments in order of strength:
  - Medial or deltoid ligament
  - Lateral ligaments (anterior and posterior talofibular, and calcaneofibular)
- Is more stable in dorsiflexion due to the broader anterior–superior surface of the talus bone
- Is innervated by the deep peroneal and tibial nerves
- Is supplied by the anterior and posterior tibial arteries.

The foot joints:

- Include the:
  - Subtalar joint where eversion and inversion occur
  - Midtarsal joints (talocalcaneonavicular and calcaneocuboid) where eversion and inversion occur

- Tarsometatarsal, intermetatarsal, metatarsophalangeal and interphalangeal joints
- Are all synovial joints except the fibrous cuboideonavicular joint.

Muscles (Figure 1.16)

The leg has a robust interosseous membrane that connects the tibia and fibula with anterior, lateral and posterior compartments divided by strong intermuscular septa:

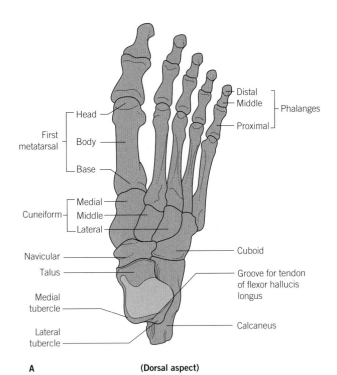

A **(Dorsal aspect)**

FIGURE 1.18

(**A**) Bony anatomy of the foot. The medial longitudinal arch includes the calcaneus, talus, navicular, three cuneiforms and the three medial metatarsals. The lateral longitudinal arch includes the calcaneus, cuboid and two lateral metatarsals. The transverse arch includes the proximal metatarsals as well as the three cuneiforms and the cuboid.

Continued

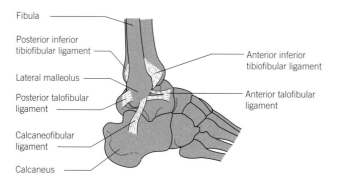

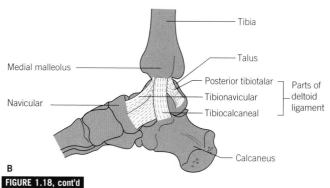

B

FIGURE 1.18, cont'd

(**B**) Ankle ligaments. The lateral ligament runs from the lateral malleolus to the calcaneus and talus (neck and lateral tubercle) bones. The medial ligament runs from the medial malleolus to the navicular (tuberosity), calcaneus (anterior–medial margin of sustentaculum tali) and talus (medial tubercle) bones.

- Anterior compartment (tibialis anterior, extensor digitorum longus, extensor hallucis longus, peroneus tertius):
  - Is innervated by the deep peroneal nerve
  - Is responsible for toe extension, foot dorsiflexion and contributions to foot inversion (tibialis anterior) and eversion (peroneus tertius) (Table 1.8)
- Lateral compartment (peroneus brevis and peroneus longus):
  - Is innervated by the superficial peroneal nerve
  - Is responsible for foot eversion and plantar flexion (Table 1.8)
- Posterior compartment (gastrocnemius, plantaris, soleus, tibialis posterior, flexor digitorum longus, flexor hallucis longus):
  - Is innervated by the tibial nerve
  - Is responsible for plantar flexion, toe flexion and foot inversion (tibialis posterior) (Tables 1.8 and 1.9)

TABLE 1.8

THE MUSCLES, WITH THEIR INNERVATIONS, WHICH PROVIDE MOVEMENT AT THE ANKLE JOINT AND FOOT (EVERSION AND INVERSION)

Movement	Muscle	Origin	Insertion	Nerve
Dorsiflexion	Extensor hallucis longus (A)	Fibula and interosseous membrane	Big toe, distal phalanx	Deep peroneal
	Extensor digitorum longus (A)	Tibia and interosseous membrane	Middle/distal phalanx (lateral four toes)	Deep peroneal
	Peroneus tertius (A)	Fibula and interosseous membrane	Fifth MT base	Deep peroneal
	Tibialis anterior (A)	Tibia and interosseous membrane	First MT base, medial cuneiform	Deep peroneal
Plantar flexion	Peroneus longus (L)	Fibula	First MT, medial cuneiform	Superficial peroneal
	Peroneus brevis (L)	Fibula	Fifth MT	Superficial peroneal
	Plantaris (PS)	Lateral supracondyle of femur	Calcaneum	Tibial
	Gastrocnemius (PS)	Posterior condyles of femur	Calcaneum (via AT)	Tibial
	Soleus (PS)	Fibula and medial border of tibia	Calcaneum (via AT)	Tibial
	Flexor digitorum longus (PD)	Posterior aspect of tibia	Distal phalanges (lateral four toes)	Tibial
	Flexor hallucis longus (PD)	Posterior aspect of fibula	Distal phalanx of big toe	Tibial
	Tibialis posterior (PD)	Tibia and fibula	Navicular, medial cuneiform	Tibial
Eversion	Peroneus tertius (A)	Anterior aspect of fibula	Fifth MT base	Deep peroneal
	Peroneus longus (L)	Fibula	First MT, medial cuneiform	Superficial peroneal
	Peroneus brevis (L)	Fibula	Fifth MT	Superficial peroneal
Inversion	Tibialis anterior (A)	Tibia and interosseous membrane	First MT base, medial cuneiform	Deep peroneal
	Tibialis posterior (PD)	Tibia and fibula	Navicular, medial cuneiform	Tibial

A, anterior compartment of leg; AT, Achilles tendon; D, deep; L, lateral compartment of leg; MT, metatarsal; P, posterior compartment of leg; S, superficial.

TABLE 1.9

THE MUSCLES, WITH THEIR INNERVATIONS, WHICH PROVIDE MOVEMENT OF THE TOES

Movement	Muscle	Origin	Insertion	Nerve
Big toe abduction	Abductor hallucis (first layer)	Calcaneum, FR, PA	Big toe, proximal phalanx	Medial plantar
Big toe adduction	Adductor hallucis (third layer)			Lateral plantar
	Oblique head	Second → fourth MT bases	Big toe, proximal phalanx	
	Transverse head	Transverse ligament	Big toe, proximal phalanx	
Big toe flexion	Flexor hallucis longus	Posterior aspect of fibula	Big toe, distal phalanx	Tibial
	Flexor hallucis brevis (third layer)	Cuboid, cuneiforms	Big toe, proximal phalanx	Medial plantar
Big toe extension	Extensor hallucis longus	Fibula and interosseous membrane	Big toe, distal phalanx	Deep peroneal
Little toe abduction	Abductor digiti minimi (first layer)	Calcaneus, PA	Fifth toe, proximal phalanx	Lateral plantar
Little toe flexion	Flexor digiti minimi brevis (third layer)	Fifth MT	Fifth toe, proximal phalanx	Medial plantar
Digital abduction	Dorsal interossei (fourth layer)	MT	Digits, proximal phalanx	Lateral plantar
Digital adduction	Plantar interossei (fourth layer)	Third–fifth MT	Digits, proximal phalanx	Lateral plantar
Digital flexion	Flexor digitorum longus	Posterior aspect of tibia	Distal phalanx (lateral four toes)	Tibial
	Flexor digitorum brevis (first layer)	Calcaneum, PA	Middle phalanx (lateral four toes)	Medial plantar
Digital extension	Extensor digitorum longus	Tibia and interosseous membrane	Middle/distal phalanx (lateral four toes)	Deep peroneal

The lumbricals are responsible for PIPJ flexion and IPJ/DIPJ extension.
FR, flexor retinaculum; MT, metatarsal; PA, plantar aponeurosis.

- Gastrocnemius and plantaris provide minor contributions to knee flexion
- The intrinsic muscles of the foot are divided into four layers and they are responsible for the movements of the toes (Table 1.9).

Blood Supply

- Anterior tibial artery supplies the anterior compartment of the leg and ankle joint:

- The origin is the popliteal artery and it starts at the inferior edge of the popliteus muscle
- It is susceptible to ischaemia due to anterior compartment syndrome
- It becomes the dorsalis pedis artery (palpable between extensor hallucis longus medially and extensor digitorum longus laterally) as it passes inferiorly to the extensor retinaculum anterior to the ankle, which supplies the foot and then forms the plantar arch (anastomosis with lateral plantar artery), which gives rise to metatarsal and digital arteries
- Posterior tibial artery supplies the posterior and lateral compartments of the leg and the ankle joint:
  - The origin is the popliteal artery and it starts at the inferior edge of the popliteus muscle
  - It runs inferior to soleus and gastrocnemius
  - It gives rise to the peroneal (fibular) artery, ~2–3 cm below popliteus, that predominantly supplies the lateral compartment of the leg
  - It becomes the medial and lateral plantar arteries (as it passes inferiorly to the flexor retinaculum), which supply the foot via their own branches and the palmar arch.

Nerves

- Common peroneal nerve (L4-L5 and S1-S2) arises after a division of the sciatic nerve just superior to the popliteal fossa (lateral to the tibial nerve), where it provides some innervation to the knee joint. It then circles the fibula neck and divides to give:
  - Sensory cutaneous divisions (sural nerve)
  - The deep peroneal nerve (passes inferiorly to the extensor retinaculum), which innervates the ankle joint and the anterior compartment of the leg, and provides sensation to the first web space of the dorsum of the foot (Figure 1.19)
  - The superficial peroneal nerve, which innervates the lateral compartment of the leg and some intrinsic muscles of the foot, and provides sensation to the anterior aspect of the leg and the dorsum of the foot (Figure 1.19)
- Tibial nerve (L4-L5 and S1-S3) arises after a division of the sciatic nerve just superior to the popliteal fossa (and superficial to popliteal vessels). It innervates the posterior compartment of the leg (running inferiorly to the soleus) as well as the ankle joint. The nerve passes posterior to the medial malleolus and then divides as it passes inferiorly to the flexor retinaculum to give:
  - The medial and lateral plantar nerves, which innervate the intrinsic muscles of the foot and provide sensory innervation to the sole of the foot (Figure 1.19)
  - Sensory cutaneous divisions (sural nerve)
- Sural cutaneous nerve (derived from the tibial and common peroneal nerves) provides sensory innervation to the posterior and lateral aspects of the leg, as well as the lateral aspect of the plantar and dorsal parts of the foot (Figure 1.19)
- Saphenous nerve (L3-L4) is the terminal branch of the femoral nerve that travels medially past the knee (posterior to sartorius), emerges between the

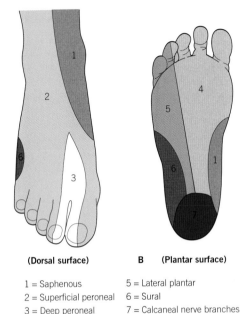

A   (Dorsal surface)   **B**   (Plantar surface)

1 = Saphenous   5 = Lateral plantar
2 = Superficial peroneal   6 = Sural
3 = Deep peroneal   7 = Calcaneal nerve branches
4 = Medial plantar

FIGURE 1.19

Sensory innervation of the foot: (**A**) dorsal and (**B**) plantar.

gracilis and sartorius tendons, and passes down the medial aspect of the leg adjacent to the great saphenous vein to provide sensory innervation to the medial aspect of the leg and ankle (Figure 1.19).

 HINTS AND TIPS

ANKLE AND FOOT

A lesion of the common peroneal nerve results in a foot drop and potentially a high stepping gait. Acute compartment syndrome following a fracture of the tibia can be associated with loss of sensation in the first dorsal web space (deep peroneal nerve/anterior compartment). The saphenous nerve and vein travel anterior to the medial malleolus and this is a site of peripheral access in a patient with shock (i.e. saphenous cut down). The mnemonic for structures that pass posterior to the medial malleolus are **T**om, **D**ick **A**nd a **N**ervous **H**arry (anterior to posterior) – **t**ibialis posterior tendon, flexor **d**igitorum longus tendon, posterior tibial **a**rtery, tibial **n**erve and flexor digitorum **h**allucis tendon. The longitudinal and transverse arches of the foot aid in weight bearing and walking.

SPINE

Bones and Joints (Figures 1.20 and 1.21)

The vertebral column begins with the cervical vertebrae below the skull (atlantooccipital joint), ending with the fused vertebrae that form the sacrum and the coccyx:

- The primary sagittal curvatures are found in the thoracic (kyphosis) and sacrococcygeal regions.
- The secondary sagittal curvatures are found in the cervical (lordosis) and lumbar (lordosis) regions.
- The thoracic kyphosis balances the cervical and lumbar lordosis.
- Spinal nerve roots comprise:
  - Eight cervical (seven vertebrae)
  - Twelve thoracic

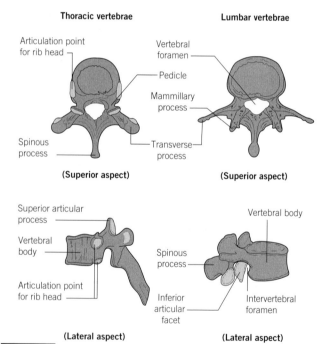

Thoracic vertebrae

Articulation point for rib head

Vertebral foramen

Pedicle

Mammillary process

Spinous process

Transverse process

(Superior aspect)

Lumbar vertebrae

(Superior aspect)

Superior articular process

Vertebral body

Articulation point for rib head

Spinous process

Inferior articular facet

(Lateral aspect)

Vertebral body

Intervertebral foramen

(Lateral aspect)

FIGURE 1.20

Characteristic features of individual vertebrae. The synovial articular facet joints provide articulation between the individual vertebrae. These joints are supported by surrounding ligaments (supra- and interspinous, anterior and posterior longitudinal, and ligamenta flava).

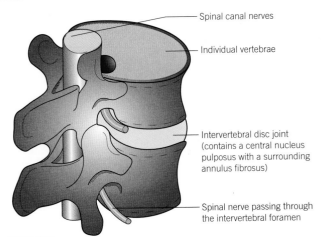

Spinal canal nerves

Individual vertebrae

Intervertebral disc joint (contains a central nucleus pulposus with a surrounding annulus fibrosus)

Spinal nerve passing through the intervertebral foramen

FIGURE 1.21

The secondary cartilaginous intervertebral disc (consists of the nucleus pulposus and annulus fibrosus) joint provides the macro-movements of the spine.

- Five lumbar
- Five sacral and one coccygeal.
- The adult spinal cord terminates at L1.
- Most vertebrae have an anterior body and a posterior ring (pedicle, lamina, lateral and posterior spinous processes):
  - Protect neural elements within the spinal canal.
- Vertebrae are separated by an intervertebral disc consisting of a nucleus pulposus within an annulus fibrosus:
  - Longitudinal ligaments also add to intervertebral strength.

Muscles of the Thoracolumbar Group (Figure 1.22)

- Extrinsic muscles of the back involve those connected with movement of the shoulder and arm (e.g. latissimus dorsi) and those connected with breathing (e.g. serratus posterior).
- The intrinsic muscles of the back are those involved with the fundamental movements of the spine (e.g. erector spinae, quadratus lumborum, psoas major). Unbalanced muscle action can lead to displacement and rotation of a section of the vertebrae, i.e. scoliosis.

Blood Supply

The anterior and two posterior spinal arteries are supplied by the vertebral, deep cervical, intercostal and lumbar arteries. In the lower spinal cord the anterior spinal artery is predominantly supplied by the radicular artery of Adamkiewicz. The blood supply of the vertebral column levels comprises:

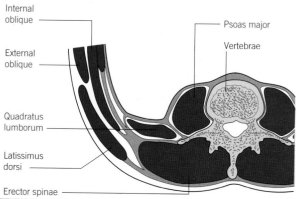

Internal oblique

Psoas major

Vertebrae

External oblique

Quadratus lumborum

Latissimus dorsi

Erector spinae

FIGURE 1.22

Muscles of the back. The erector spinae muscles are involved in spinal flexion and extension, as well as lateral flexion. Not shown are the transversospinalis muscles that are involved in spinal extension and rotation, and the intertransversarii and interspinales muscles that are involved in spinal extension and lateral flexion.

- Cervical, e.g. vertebral or basilar arteries
- Thoracic, e.g. intercostal or anterior spinal arteries
- Lumbar, e.g. lumbar segmental or common iliac arteries
- Sacral, e.g. internal iliac or sacral arteries.

HINTS AND TIPS

SPINE

With increasing years the intervertebral disc will dry out and degenerate (which can lead to back pain). The nucleus pulposus can herniate through the annulus fibrosus (a slipped disc). This can in turn lead to compression of the sciatic nerve roots, which may lead to pain and paraesthesia down the leg (sciatica), with motor involvement also possible, e.g. weakness of big toe extension. The most commonly affected levels are L4-L5 and L5-S1.

Chapter 2
History and Examination

History (Figure 2.1) and clinical examination should always start with an introduction to the patient, giving your name and role. It is then important to confirm identification of the patient, usually by asking their name and date of birth, followed by an explanation of what is about to be done and obtaining the patient's verbal consent to proceed.

Clinical examination (Figure 2.1) in orthopaedics and rheumatology routinely follows a 'triad' system, developed by Graham Apley, of look/inspect, feel and move. Special tests and a complete neurovascular examination should then follow as indicated. It is important to remember that inspection commences as soon as the patient enters the room. Gait, the use of walking aids and any evidence that they are in pain as they move can provide useful information before the consultation begins.

A good clinical examination should maintain the dignity of the patient but requires adequate exposure of the joint above and below the affected region along with the contralateral side for comparison. On inspection, the main aspects are the skin (e.g. for scars, erythema, rashes, bruising and stigmata of disease), the soft tissues (e.g. for effusions, joint swelling, masses, wasting) and then the overall alignment and configuration of the skeleton (e.g. varus or valgus, fixed flexion deformity, kyphosis or scoliosis). Before progressing to feel it is important to ascertain whether the patient is in pain and to watch the patient's face to determine if they are in any discomfort. Movement requires both active (by the patient) and passive (by the examiner) assessment. Important nomenclature includes:

- Abduction (away from midline) and adduction (towards midline)
- Flexion (forward/anterior movement of trunk/limb) and extension (backwards/posterior)
- Internal (medial) rotation (rotation towards/medial midline) and external (lateral) rotation (rotation away/lateral from midline)
- Pronation–supination (palms/soles down/posterior and palms/soles up/anterior)
- Inversion–eversion (foot moves medial–lateral).

In some patients, the range of joint movement may exceed the normal expected limits. If this is found, formal testing should be performed for hypermobility (Table 2.1). A Beighton score of 6 or more is indicative of joint hypermobility.

When assessing sensation the stroke test compared to the contralateral side can be used, but for accurate detailing of the sensory abnormality, two-point discrimination may be required. Muscle power can be graded using the Medical Research Council (MRC) scale (Table 2.2). It is important to understand the action of each muscle, as well as the nerve root(s) and the peripheral nerve(s) that innervate it.

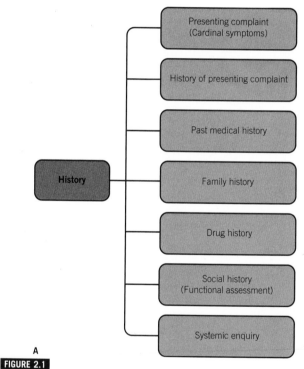

A

FIGURE 2.1

The algorithm for history (**A**) and examination (**B**) of the musculoskeletal system. On physical examination, the headings Inspect, Feel, Move and Special tests comprise a logical order. Remember to assess gait in lower limb and spine disorders. Please see Figure 2.20 and Table 2.5 for details of the neurological assessment of the upper and lower limbs.

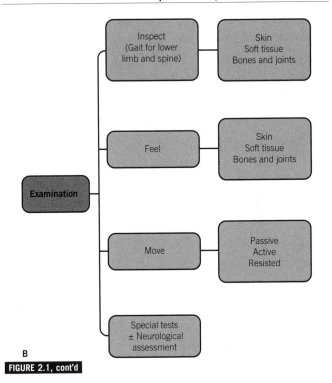

B

FIGURE 2.1, cont'd

TABLE 2.1

THE BEIGHTON SCORE FOR HYPERMOBILITY

Test	Score*
Hyperextend little finger >90° at MCP joint	1 point for each side
Bring thumb back to touch the flexor surface of the forearm	1 point for each side
Hyperextend elbow >10°	1 point for each side
Hyperextend knee >10°	1 point for each side
Touch the floor with the flat of the hands with knees straight	1 point

*A score of 6 or more indicates hypermobility.

HISTORY

Presenting Complaint

Where possible a concise description of the problem should be obtained (e.g. injured left ankle, painful left hip, generalized joint pain and swelling).

TABLE 2.2

THE MRC GRADING OF POWER AS PART OF THE NEUROLOGICAL ASSESSMENT

Grade	Description
0	No contraction
1	Contraction traceable
2	Full range of active movement with gravity eliminated
3	Full range of active movement against gravity
4	Reduced power on active movement against resistance
4+	Detectable minimal reduction in power against resistance
5	Full and normal power against resistance

History of Presenting Complaint

Ask the patient to recall when the primary symptom started and describe what it was like. Things to enquire about include:

- Sudden *vs.* gradual onset
- Single *vs.* multiple joints
- Small *vs.* large joints
- Precipitating factors, e.g. infection, medications and trauma
- When the presentation is with pain, use the mnemonic **SOCRATES** to describe the key characteristics: **s**ite, **o**nset, **c**haracter, **r**adiation, **a**lleviating factors, **t**iming, **e**xacerbating factors and **s**everity
- Ask about swelling, redness and heat
- Ask about systemic symptoms:
  - Malaise, weight loss or anorexia
- Ask about early-morning stiffness (suggests inflammatory cause)
- Ask if the symptoms are worse on movement (suggests mechanical pathology), or paradoxically worse when resting (non-mechanical)
- Ask about the functional consequences:
  - Effects on activities of daily living and occupation
- Ask about muscle weakness
- Proximal *vs.* distal.

Red flag symptoms of back pain are important potential indicators of significant pathology (e.g. infection, tumour, spinial cord or cauda equina compression):

- Sudden onset of back pain
- Recent significant trauma
- Previous malignant disease
- Systemic symptoms (e.g. unexplained weight loss and fever)
- Immunosuppressives (e.g. corticosteroids, DMARDs, biological drugs)
- Severe or progressive neurological (sensory and/or motor) changes
- Painless urinary retention
- Paraesthesia in the perineum or buttocks and/or faecal incontinence.

Past Medical History

It is important to enquire about previously diagnosed rheumatological disorders, such as RA, vasculitis, SLE, OA and osteoporosis. Similarly, it is important to determine if there have been any episodes of trauma in the past, including previous surgical procedures for musculoskeletal conditions. For all patients it is essential to document any history of developmental delay or joint problems, including infection during childhood, along with any previous surgery. The patient should be asked about other major illnesses including:

- Cardiovascular and cerebrovascular disease
- Previous pulmonary embolus (PE) or deep venous thrombosis (DVT) including a family history of coagulopathy
- Diabetes and other endocrine diseases
- Chronic obstructive airways disease or asthma
- Epilepsy
- Gastrointestinal disease
- Chronic kidney disease
- Immunosuppressive disease e.g. HIV/AIDS
- Medications (see Drug History).

Family History

Many musculoskeletal disorders have an inherited component and a positive family history may be obtained in:

- Rheumatological conditions, e.g. RA, psoriatic arthritis, ankylosing spondylitis, SLE, gout
- Hypermobility syndrome (Table 2.1)
- Osteoporosis
- Congenital skeletal abnormalities, e.g. developmental dysplasia of the hip
- Some primary bone tumours and tumour-like conditions, e.g. neurofibromatosis
- Haematological disorders, e.g. haemophilia
- Skeletal dysplasias e.g. fibrous dysplasia and dwarfism.

Drug History (see Chapter 8)

Important medications to enquire about are:

- Analgesia:
  - NSAIDs due to the risk of gastrointestinal bleeding and renal impairment
  - Opioids due to potential side effects and tolerance; also a useful marker of pain severity in most cases
- Anticoagulation:
  - Aspirin, clopidogrel, warfarin and novel oral anticoagulants (e.g. rivaroxaban)
  - The use of these drugs indicates a history of cardiovascular or thromboembolic disease and they may need to be adjusted or temporarily stopped perioperatively (Chapters 4 and 8)

- Corticosteroids, as long-term use predisposes to osteoporosis and infections, along with numerous other side effects
- Diuretics, particularly thiazides, are common precipitants in gout
- Minocycline, hydralazine and procainamide are potential precipitants of drug-induced lupus
- DMARDs which have a large number of potential side effects
- Biologicals that cause immunosuppression:
  - Usually should be stopped preoperatively
- Over-the-counter medications including herbal remedies
- Drug allergies.

Social History

A full assessment should be performed, including:

- Occupation, including partner's
- Living environment (apartment, house, number of stairs)
- Family dynamics:
  - Is there a disabled elderly parent or spouse to look after?
  - What about children? Are they nearby to help if an operation with prolonged recovery is contemplated?
- Activities of daily living:
  - Normal mobility and the use of any aids
  - Washing, dressing, walking (stairs), writing and meal preparation
  - Social support, e.g. carers
- Alcohol consumption
- Smoking and recreational drugs
- Diet.

Systemic Enquiry

In addition to a systematic enquiry covering the cardiovascular, respiratory, gastrointestinal, genitourinary and neurological systems the following features should be specifically asked about:

- Systemic upset: fevers, sweats, malaise and weight loss:
  - May indicate infection, vasculitis or occult malignancy
- Breathlessness:
  - Consider pulmonary fibrosis or cardiac involvement in vasculitis, SLE or connective tissue disease (CTD)
- Pitting of nails and onycholysis:
  - Suggests psoriatic arthritis
- Skin rash on extensor surfaces:
  - Suggests psoriatic arthritis
- Photosensitive rash:
  - Suggests SLE
- Dry mouth or gritty eyes:
  - Suggests Sjögren syndrome
- Painful or red eyes:
  - Consider uveitis or conjunctivitis
- Mouth ulcers:
  - Consider SLE or Behçet syndrome

- Recurrent miscarriages:
  - Suggests SLE or antiphospholipid syndrome.

 HINTS AND TIPS

HISTORY

The key aspects of a good history start with a clear presenting complaint and the details of this, along with any associated symptoms. Red flag symptoms, which usually indicate a significant underlying pathology, include non-mechanical pain, night pain, appetite and weight loss, fever, malaise and night sweats. The past medical and drug history should include a childhood history and previous surgery. A relevant family history will aid with the diagnosis and highlight potential risk factors. The social history should include details on smoking, alcohol, occupation, the level of mobility and the use of walking aids, along with activities of daily living and the use of social support.

WRIST AND HAND

Inspect

- Skin and nail alterations:
  - Onycholysis and pitting in psoriatic patients
  - Nail infarcts and ulcers in vasculitis
  - Red scaly rash on extensor surfaces in psoriatic arthritis
- Photosensitive rash in SLE
- Raynaud symptoms in SLE and CTD
- Skin thickening in scleroderma and CTD
- Muscle wasting (note if unilateral or bilateral):
  - Thenar eminence (median nerve)
  - Hypothenar eminence (ulnar nerve)
  - Interosseous muscles (intermetacarpal recession on dorsum of hand sometimes seen in RA or an ulnar nerve lesion)
- Swelling, redness and heat of a single joint:
  - Indicative of gout, pseudogout, infection or reactive arthritis
- Soft tissue swelling of multiple joints:
  - Indicative of RA, PsA and seronegative spondyloarthropathy
- Bony swelling of the PIPJ and DIPJ:
  - OA
- Swelling of tendons and tendon sheaths:
  - Indicative of RA, infection and other inflammatory diseases
- Deformities:
  - Subluxations and fractures
  - Bone deformity in Paget disease
  - Swan neck, boutonnière, nodules, ulnar deviation and Z-thumb deformity in RA (see Chapter 5)
  - Heberden and Bouchard nodes in OA (see Chapter 5)
  - Tophi in gout
  - Sclerodactyly (diabetes, scleroderma, SLE)
  - Thickening of the palmar fascia with a fixed flexion deformity of the finger (Dupuytren contracture).

Feel

- Bony tenderness:
  - Fracture (e.g. anatomical snuff box in the suspected scaphoid fracture)
  - Enthesitis (e.g. tendon insertions in ankylosing spondylitis)
  - Osteomalacia (generalized bone tenderness)
- Soft tissue swelling:
  - Periarticular tenderness and warmth suggests synovitis or infection
- Flexor tendon (sheaths) for swelling and thickening
- Sensation in the ulnar, radial and median nerve dermatomes (see Chapter 1, Figure 1.12)
- Crepitus or trigger finger on joint movement.

Move

- Ask about pain on movement
- Pinch strength, precision pinch and grip strength
- Wrist radial deviation 0–25°, ulnar deviation 0–50°, dorsiflexion/extension 0–90° (Figure 2.2) and flexion 0–90° (Figure 2.3)
- MCPJ, PIPJ and DIPJ flexion and extension
- Hyperextension of digits (may indicate hypermobility – Table 2.1)
- Specific muscles and the nerve supply are detailed in Table 2.3.

Special Tests

- Finkelstein test (De Quervain tenosynovitis, see Chapter 6)
- Tinel and Phalen test:
  - Carpal tunnel syndrome, see Chapter 6
  - Ulnar nerve pathology
- Froment sign (Figure 2.4):
  - Ulnar nerve pathology
- Allen test:
  - Assesses contribution of radial and ulnar arteries to palmar arch
  - Occlude both arteries at the wrist with palpation

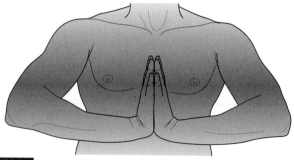

FIGURE 2.2
Wrist extension (the prayer sign).

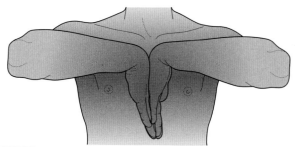

Wrist flexion.

TABLE 2.3

ASSESSMENT OF THE MUSCLES AND NERVES OF THE HAND AND WRIST

Finger PIPJ flexion is assessed by holding the other fingers in fixed extension and asking the patient to flex the finger being examined. To assess finger DIPJ flexion hold the PIPJ in fixed extension for the finger being examined. Extensor digitorum communis is supplied by the radial nerve posterior interosseous branch and contributes to extension of hand, wrist and fingers (but remember that the lumbricals and interossei can also extend the IP joints while flexing the MCP joint)

Movement	Muscle	Innervation
Thumb abduction	Abductor pollicis brevis	Median nerve
	Abductor pollicis longus	Radial nerve (PIN)
Thumb adduction	Adductor pollicis	Ulnar nerve
Thumb flexion:		
MCPJ	Flexor pollicis brevis	Median nerve
IPJ	Flexor pollicis longus	Median nerve (AIN)
Thumb extension:		
MCPJ	Extensor pollicis brevis	Radial nerve (PIN)
IPJ	Extensor pollicis longus	Radial nerve (PIN)
Finger abduction	Dorsal interossei	Ulnar nerve
Finger adduction	Palmar interossei	Ulnar nerve
Finger flexion:		
PIPJ	Flexor digitorum superficialis	Median nerve
DIPJ (index, middle)	Flexor digitorum profundus	Median nerve (AIN)
DIPJ (ring, little)	Flexor digitorum profundus	Ulnar nerve
Wrist extension and abduction	Extensor carpi radialis longus	Radial nerve
	Extensor carpi radialis brevis	Radial nerve (PIN)
Wrist extension and adduction	Extensor carpi ulnaris	Radial nerve (PIN)
Wrist flexion and abduction	Flexor carpi radialis	Median nerve
Wrist flexion and adduction	Flexor carpi ulnaris	Ulnar nerve

PIN: posterior interosseous nerve.

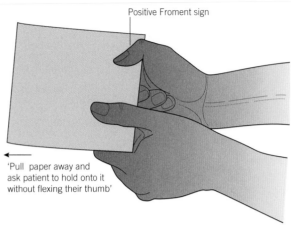

Positive Froment sign

'Pull paper away and
ask patient to hold onto it
without flexing their thumb'

FIGURE 2.4

Froment sign. The patient cannot hold onto the paper when it is pulled away without
flexion of the right thumb IPJ (flexor pollis longus/brevis – median nerve) due to a
weakness of right thumb adduction (adductor pollicis – ulnar nerve).

- Patient makes a fist several times until the hand goes pale
- Release each artery in turn to assess re-perfusion of hand.

> **💡 HINTS AND TIPS**
>
> **WRIST AND HAND**
>
> You can learn a lot on inspection of the hands and wrists. The distribution of
> joint involvement is often enough to point you in the direction of RA
> (symmetrically affecting the wrists, MCPJ and PIPJ), OA (PIPJ, DIPJ, first CMCJ)
> or PsA (asymmetrically affecting the DIPJ and PIPJ with nail dystrophy and
> rash). Patients with RA are often difficult to assess formally for range of
> movement and it can be helpful to assess some generic movements such as
> writing and doing a button-up. A concise neurological assessment of the hand
> includes the median nerve (sensation in the radial 3.5 digits, power of thumb
> abduction), anterior interosseous nerve ('OK sign' with assessment of the flexor
> pollicis longus and index FDP), ulnar nerve (sensation in the ulnar one and half
> digits, power of little finger abduction) and the radial nerve (sensation in the first
> dorsal web space, power of thumb extension).

ELBOW AND FOREARM

Inspect

- Swelling, redness and heat:
  - Olecranon bursitis (RA)
  - Psoriatic plaques on extensor surfaces
  - Effusion (often found in the lateral infracondylar space)

- Deformities:
  - Joints (RA, OA, infection)
  - Tendons and tendon sheaths (RA)
  - Nodules (RA)
  - Fracture and/or dislocation
  - Disturbance of normal carrying angle:
    - Axis of upper arm to forearm
    - Patient stands with elbows in full extension and forearm supinated
    - Normal ~7–16° (and greater in women than men)
    - Abnormal, e.g. cubitus varus after a supracondylar fracture
  - Muscle wasting.

Feel

- Regional tenderness or temperature:
  - Epicondyles (golfer's/medial and tennis/lateral elbow)
  - Lateral and medial collateral ligament complexes
- Olecranon:
  - Nodules (RA), effusion and tophi
- Crepitus on joint movement, including radial head on supination and pronation.

Move

- Ask if any pain on movement
- Flexion and extension (0–150°)
- Pronation (0–90°) and supination (0–90°) with elbows flexed to 90° and shoulders adducted
- Collateral ligaments with arm in extension and in approximately 25° of flexion:
  - Assess for varus–valgus instability.

Special Tests

- Lateral epicondylitis (tennis elbow):
  - Pain on resisted wrist and finger extension
- Medial epicondylitis (golfer's elbow):
  - Pain on resisted wrist and finger flexion
- Tinel test:
  - Ulnar nerve pathology.

 HINTS AND TIPS

ELBOW AND FOREARM

A functional arc of motion in the elbow is thought to be from 30° of extension to 130° of flexion. A classic claw appearance to the hand (due to intrinsic muscle weakness) can occur when a lesion to the ulnar nerve occurs at the wrist, e.g. in the Guyon canal. However, the ulnar paradox occurs when the pathology is more proximal at the elbow, with the clawing less severe due to loss of innervation of the FDP muscle to the ring and little fingers.

SHOULDER

Inspect

- Anterior and posterior:
  - Shoulder contour symmetry
- Muscle wasting:
  - Frozen shoulder
  - Rotator cuff pathology
  - Neurological disorder
- Swelling, redness and heat:
  - Effusion, which may be hidden by the deltoid muscle
- Deformities:
  - Scapula winging (e.g. long thoracic nerve palsy)
  - Dislocation (acromioclavicular joint or glenohumeral 'step')
  - Prominent acromioclavicular or sternoclavicular joint (OA and/or previous injury).

Feel

- Joint and soft tissue tenderness and/or swelling at the:
  - Acromioclavicular, sternoclavicular and glenohumeral joints
  - Clavicle (check for deformity or evidence of instability)
  - Shoulder point and subacromial space
  - Scapular spine
- Crepitus on joint movement
- Sensation over the axillary nerve cutaneous innervation (regimental badge sign).

Move

- Ask if any pain on movement
- Hands behind head and push elbows back (Figure 2.5A):
  - Assess shoulder flexion, abduction and external (lateral) rotation
- Hands together behind back (Figure 2.5B):
  - Assess shoulder extension, adduction and internal (medial) rotation
- Specific movements of the shoulder joint:
  - Internal rotation (finger tips to reach T4-T9 spinous processes) and external rotation (0–50°) with the elbow flexed to 90° and the shoulder in full adduction (Figure 2.6A)
  - Flexion (180°) and extension (60°) using a hand on the blade of the scapula to immobilize it (Figure 2.6B)
  - Abduction (180°) and adduction (30°) using a hand on the blade of the scapula to immobilize it (Figure 2.7). The first 60–80° of abduction is due to the glenohumeral joint alone, whereas beyond this point both glenohumeral and scapulothoracic joints are responsible for abduction.

Special Tests

- Rotator cuff:
  - Painful abduction against resistance may indicate supraspinatus tendon inflammation

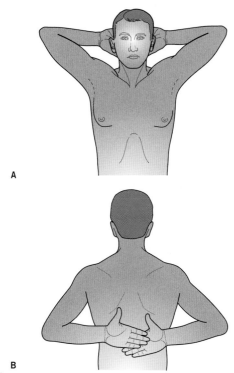

A

B

An overall assessment of shoulder movements. (**A**) Hands behind head with elbows pushed back. (**B**) Hands behind back with elbows pushed back. *(Adapted from Ford et al 2005.)*

- Active initiation of abduction is possible, then pain between 40° and 120° = painful arc syndrome (Figure 2.8), which is seen in rotator cuff impingement; symptoms reproduced when shoulder is abducted to ~100° and internally rotated (Hawkins test for supraspinatus impingement)
- Passive abduction to 30–45°, active abduction thereafter (due to deltoid) = rotator cuff (supraspinatus) rupture:
  - Jobe sign with arm abducted to 90° and forward to 30°, internal rotation with thumbs pointing to the floor, push down on the arm
  - Weakness and or pain is indicative of a tear or impingement
- Pain on resisted internal rotation is indicative of subscapularis pathology (Gerber test to confirm = unable to lift the back of the hand away from the spine when requested)
- Pain on resisted external rotation is indicative of infraspinatus pathology

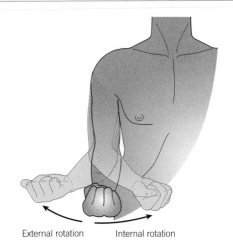

A   External rotation   Internal rotation

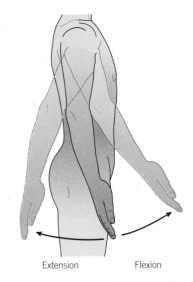

B   Extension   Flexion

FIGURE 2.6

Movements of the shoulder joint. (**A**) External and internal rotation of the shoulder. External rotation loss may indicate frozen shoulder, OA or shoulder dislocation. Pain on resisted external rotation may indicate infraspinatus pathology. Pain on resisted internal rotation may indicate subscapularis pathology. (**B**) Flexion and extension of the shoulder. *(Adapted from Ford et al 2005.)*

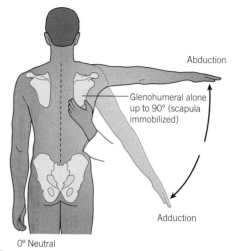

FIGURE 2.7

Abduction and adduction of the shoulder.

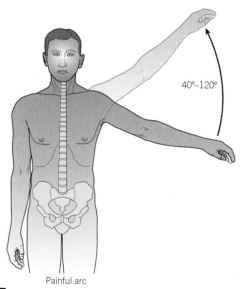

FIGURE 2.8

Painful arc syndrome may indicate subacromial impingement. However, a painful arc towards the vertical (160–180°) may indicate acromioclavicular pathology and can be reinforced by a positive scarf test (pain over ACJ when arm forward elevated to 90 degrees and actively adducted across chest). *(Adapted from Ford et al 2005.)*

- Brachial plexus assessment:
  - Motor and sensory assessment can be guided using Figure 2.20 and Table 2.5
- Yergason test:
  - Forearm supination against resistance indicative of biceps tendon inflammation
- Scapular winging test:
  - Push against wall, scapula becomes prominent
  - Medial winging – injury of long thoracic nerve (C5-C7) to serratus anterior, e.g. during lymph node resection in axilla or perhaps due to a mononeuritis
  - Lateral winging – trapezius weakness (spinal accessory nerve).

 HINTS AND TIPS

SHOULDER

Neck pain can be referred to the shoulder and a full assessment of the neck is often required in patients presenting with shoulder pain. Rotator cuff problems are very common and it is important to understand how to differentiate between rupture and inflammation, with the former not always associated with pain but a reduced range of movement and loss of function. In frozen shoulder, glenohumeral movement is markedly impaired with pathognomonic loss of external rotation. Winging of the scapula can occur either medially (due to weakness of the serratus anterior) or laterally (due to weakness of the trapezius).

HIP

Inspect

- Gait to look at rhythm and symmetry (Table 2.4):
  - Trendelenburg (waddling or rolling) gait is due to dysfunction of the pelvic abductors, thus not raising the pelvis on the weight-bearing side when walking
  - Trendelenburg test (Figure 2.9) may be positive with weak gluteal abductors, e.g. developmental dysplasia of the hip, coxa vara, polio, hip dislocation or femoral neck deformities, and postsurgical
  - Antalgic gait is a pain-reducing gait as the patient attempts to decrease the duration of weight bearing on the affected hip, by means of a unilateral short stride
  - Drop foot gait is due to weak dorsiflexor muscles of the ankle and involves a high-stepping knee with toe planting, e.g. in a common peroneal palsy
- Standing:
  - Scoliosis, kyphosis and loss of lumbar lordosis
  - Pelvic obliquity
- Supine:
  - Check pelvis is 'square' (at right angles) to spine
  - Swelling (effusion), redness, heat and muscle wasting, e.g. gluteal, deformity and surgical scars

TABLE 2.4

COMMON GAIT DISORDERS

Gait	Description	Causes
Trendelenburg	Rolling, swaying or waddling gait Gluteal abductor dysfunction (weak)	Developmental dysplasia of the hip, coxa vara, polio, previous hip surgery, L5 radiculopathy
Antalgic	Dot–dash gait Shortened period on affected limb Pain-reducing gait	OA
Broad-based	Due to lack of balance Disordered rhythm	Cerebellar ataxia, alcohol intoxication, medications, stroke, peripheral neuropathy
Drop-foot	High stepping gait High knee flexion with toe contact Weak dorsiflexors	Common peroneal neuropathy Loss of proprioception
Deformity	In-toeing Tripping gait – foot catches on weight-bearing limb	Persistent femoral anteversion

Reproduced from Table 33.3 in Datta PK, Bulstrode CJK, Nixon IJ. MCQs and EMQs in Surgery: A Bailey & Love Revision Guide. 2nd edition. CRC Press; 2015.

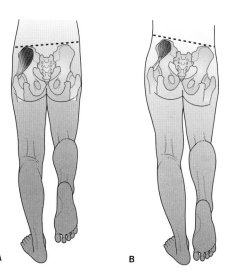

A   B

FIGURE 2.9

Trendelenburg test. Kneel down in front of the patient with your hands on their anterior superior iliac spines. Request the patient to lift each leg in turn by bending it at the knee, thus weight bearing on one leg. (**A**) Normal abductor function of the left leg, so that the left side of the pelvis tilts down and the right side rises. (**B**) Deficient abductor function of the left leg, so that the left side of the pelvis rises and the right lowers.

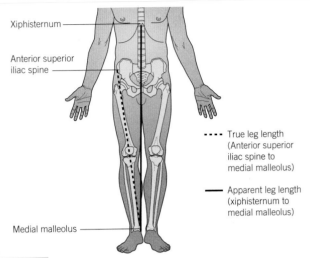

Xiphisternum

Anterior superior iliac spine

- - - - True leg length (Anterior superior iliac spine to medial malleolus)

―― Apparent leg length (xiphisternum to medial malleolus)

Medial malleolus

FIGURE 2.10

True and apparent leg length measurement. *(Adapted from Ford et al 2005.)*

- Fixed flexion deformity (FFD) using Thomas test: patient supine, place hand under lumbar lordosis and flex the unaffected normal hip until the lordosis flattens-out → FFD of affected hip becomes apparent.

Feel

- Joint, bone and soft tissue tenderness or swelling:
  - Pelvis (e.g. anterior and posterior superior iliac spines)
  - Greater trochanter (bursitis)
- Leg length measured with patient supine, pelvis square and legs flat and in the same abduction angle (Figure 2.10):
  - True: anterior superior iliac spine to medial malleolus
  - Apparent: xiphisternum to medial malleolus
- Galeazzi test:
  - Patient supine, hips at 60° flexion and knees at 90° flexion
  - Confirms leg length discrepancy at either tibia or femur.

Move

- Ask if any pain on movement
- Hip flexion 0–120° (supine) and extension 20° (prone)
- Patient and pelvis stabilized by placing arm over contralateral anterior superior iliac spine:
  - Abduction 0–50° (in adult), adduction 0–30° (Figure 2.11)

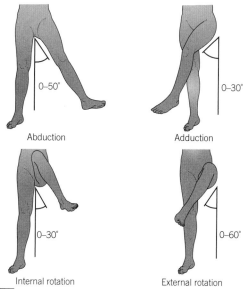

0–50°

Abduction

0–30°

Adduction

0–30°

Internal rotation

0–60°

External rotation

FIGURE 2.11

Hip abduction and adduction. Hip external and internal rotation. Decreased abduction and internal rotation may indicate OA of the hip. *(Adapted from Ford et al 2005.)*

- Patient supine with hip and knee flexed to 90°:
  - Internal rotation 0–30°, external rotation 0–60° (in adult) (Figure 2.11)
  - If pain is overwhelming, rotation of the leg with the patient lying flat on the bed will give an indication of an irritable hip
  - Femoroacetabular impingement can be assessed by flexion of the hip to ≥90°, adduction and internal rotation.

 HINTS AND TIPS

HIP

A good assessment of a patient's gait will readily assist in diagnosis, and further direct your clinical examination. Ensure overall lower limb alignment is assessed with the patient supine and weight bearing. Internal and external rotation is often reduced before flexion and extension in hip OA, with obliteration of internal rotation characteristic.

KNEE

Inspect

- Gait and standing deformities:
  - Fixed flexion deformity
  - Valgus (distance between medial malleoli, i.e. genu valgum)

- Varus (distance between medial condyles of femur, i.e. genu varum)
- Recurvatum (extension deformity) or procurvatum (flexion deformity)
- Muscle wasting:
  - Quadriceps: if notable, measure left and right thigh circumference 10 cm above each patella
- Swelling, redness and heat:
  - Anterior and posterior inspection
  - Anterior effusion (horseshoe shape) superior to knee
  - Surgical scars, e.g. midline incision and arthroscopy portals
- Supine deformities:
  - Bony contours
  - Knee alignment
  - Recurvatum or procurvatum when straight leg passively elevated off the bed.

Feel

- Joint line and ligament tenderness (with knee flexed to 90°).
- Swelling:
  - Posteriorly in the popliteal fossa (Baker cyst)
  - Prepatellar bursitis (housemaid's knee)
  - Infrapatellar bursitis (clergyman's knee)
- Effusion:
  - Bulge or Sweep test: with the patient supine and knee extended, press with four fingers on the medial aspect of the knee, below the patella, and sweep in an upward direction to remove fluid from the anteromedial compartment of the knee. Wait a few moments then repeat the action, but this time sweep down over the lateral aspect of the knee. If fluid is present you will observe a bulge on the medial aspect of the knee as fluid is displaced back into the medial compartment
  - Patellar tap (Figure 2.12): with the knee extended, remove fluid from the suprapatellar pouch as shown, then push down on the patella and a palpable 'tap' should be felt due to fluid displaced under the patella
- Crepitus on joint movement

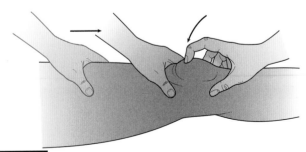

FIGURE 2.12
Testing for an effusion using the patellar tap test. *(Adapted from Ford et al 2005.)*

- Patella apprehension when passively moved laterally
- Redness and/or heat.

Move

- Ask if any pain on movement
- Knee extension and flexion (0–140°)
- Test cruciate and collateral ligaments (Figure 2.13):
  - Laxity of collateral ligament in extension is indicative of a concordant cruciate ligament injury; the collaterals are isolated at ~10–20° of knee flexion
  - Injury can be graded as normal, tender but no laxity, laxity but with a firm endpoint, laxity with no endpoint.

Special Tests

- Lachman test is an alternative for ACL instability (knee flexed to 20°, one hand on thigh and one hand behind the tibia with the thumb on the tibial tuberosity, pull tibia anteriorly)
- Pivot shift test:
  - Assess for ACL deficient knee
  - Difficult to perform unless patient deeply relaxed or anaesthetized
- McMurray test for meniscal injury (click or pain at the joint line while extending and internally/externally rotating the foot)
- Straight leg raise for extensor mechanism weakness and/or rupture (see Chapter 6):
  - Raise leg passively first to ensure full extension is attainable
  - Then patient performs actively
- Dial test is performed with patient prone and their knees flexed at 30° and 90°:
  - External rotation of both feet, positive when difference between legs is >10°
  - Positive at 30° = posterolateral corner injury
  - Positive at 90° = posterolateral corner and PCL combined injury.

 HINTS AND TIPS

KNEE

As with all joints, comparing the findings on one knee with the contralateral side can be extremely helpful. The patellar tap is only present in the case of a large effusion and the bulge test is much more sensitive and can detect small amounts of fluid. Florid crepitus over the patella on flexion of the knee is very suggestive of patellofemoral OA. When a coronal deformity is associated with OA of the knee, it is important to know if this is passively correctable or represents a fixed deformity.

ANKLE AND FOOT

Inspect

- Gait (Table 2.4) and standing deformities:
  - Assess from the side, as well as the front and back
  - Fixed equinus (may indicate neurological disorder or short limb)

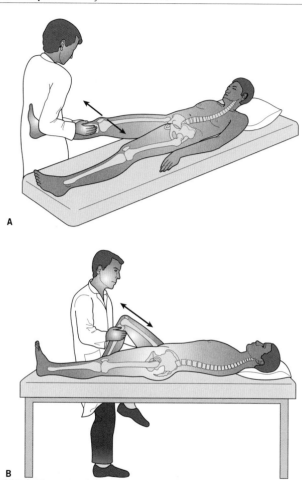

A

B

FIGURE 2.13

(**A**) The collateral ligaments are tested with the knee both fully extended and in ~10–20° degrees of flexion. Varus and valgus positional pressure on the knee tests the lateral and medial collateral ligaments. (**B**) The anterior draw test involves flexing the knee to ~90° and pulling the tibia forward (ACL). The posterior draw test involves flexing the knee to ~90° and pushing the tibia backwards (PCL). The examiner sits adjacent to the patient's foot with both hands placed on the flexed knee as shown in (**B**). *(Adapted from Ford et al 2005.)*

- Hindfoot: varus or valgus:
  - Hindfoot should normally move from valgus (on stance) to varus (on tiptoe)
- Forefoot: adduction or abduction
- Medial plantar arch: place hand in arch of foot:
  - High (pes cavus) is indicative of a neurological disorder, e.g. Charcot–Marie–Tooth disease (cavovarus foot)
  - Low (pes planus), if rigid, may indicate tarsal coalition or tibialis posterior insufficiency (too many toes sign) that can be isolated or associated with other pathologies (planovalgus foot)
- Toes: mallet, hammer and claw (Figure 2.14).
- Supine deformities:
  - Nails: clubbing or pitting
  - Skin: callosities and athletes foot

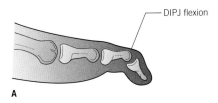

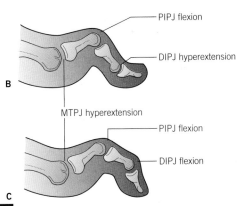

FIGURE 2.14

Deformities of the foot: (**A**) mallet toe; (**B**) hammer toe affects the middle toes most commonly; (**C**) claw toe often due to weakness of the lumbrical and interosseous muscles. The latter two are associated with hallux valgus or poor-fitting shoes. Surgical intervention may be required if conservation treatment is ineffective. *(Adapted from Coote A, Haslam P. Crash Course: Rheumatology and Orthopaedics. 2nd edition. Mosby; 2004.)*

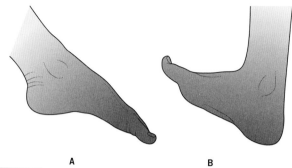

A   **B**

FIGURE 2.15

Ankle plantar flexion (**A** – push the accelerator) and dorsiflexion (**B** – release the accelerator). NB: dorsiflexion is greater with the knee flexed due to relaxation of the gastrocnemius muscle.

- Swelling, redness and heat, e.g. gout of the big toe
- Great toe abnormalities: bunion with hallux valgus, hallux rigidus.

Feel

- Joint and soft tissue tenderness, crepitus, heat and swelling:
  - Forefoot (e.g. MTPJs), midfoot (e.g. navicular) and hindfoot (e.g. malleoli, talus, Achilles)
  - Tenderness along and over the insertion of tibialis posterior (medial cuneiform and navicular).

Move

- Dorsiflexion (0–10°) and plantar flexion (0–30°) (Figure 2.15):
  - Predominantly ankle joint (test with knee flexed to relax gastrocnemius)
- Test subtalar joint movement:
  - Stabilize ankle and invert/evert calcaneus
- Test midtarsal movement:
  - Stabilize heel and pronate/supinate (midtarsal movements)
- Test for strength and discomfort of tibialis posterior, tibialis anterior and peroneal muscles (Table 1.8).

Special Tests

- Mulder sign:
  - Morton neuroma
  - Patient supine, pressure in interdigital space (usually second or third) and compression of metatarsal heads leads to characteristic pain and a click
- Silfverskiold test:
  - Ankle dorsiflexion with knee extended and knee flexed (relax gastrocnemius) to test relative contribution of a tight gastrocnemius

- Thompson or Simmonds test (see Chapter 6):
  - Patient prone with both feet hanging off the end of the bed
  - Squeeze midcalf region and look for plantar flexion
  - Achilles tendon rupture = no plantar flexion is seen
  - A step may be palpable where rupture has occurred
- Discriminate rigid (pathological) from flexible flat foot:
  - Tiptoe stance (windlass test)
  - Plantar arch should accentuate in flexible flat foot, and hindfoot moves into varus
- Neurological assessment:
  - Sensory distribution (Figure 1.19)
  - Loss of sensation in glove and stocking distribution, and not dermatomal distribution, may indicate diabetes or vitamin/folate deficiency
- Vascular assessment:
  - Assess for the dorsal pedis and posterior tibial pulses
  - Doppler and ankle brachial pressure index (ABPI) can be useful.

 HINTS AND TIPS

ANKLE AND FOOT

Inspection standing and supine is important when defining foot and ankle deformities. Always remember to assess for callosities as this may indicate an area of excessive weight bearing and can point to the underling pathology. Subluxation of the metatarsal heads with clawing of the digits is typical of advanced RA.

SPINE

Inspect

- Muscle wasting
- Swelling, redness or heat (unusual)
- From the back (coronal plane) and the side (sagittal plane) for deformities (Figure 2.16):
  - Torticollis in the neck (coronal)
  - Kyphosis (sagittal):
    - Normal thoracic kyphosis (20–50°)
    - Increases with advancing age
  - Scoliosis (coronal):
    - Muscle spasm may mimic a local scoliosis
  - Lordosis (sagittal):
    - Cervical lordosis (20–45°)
    - Lumbar lordosis (40–80°), predominantly between L4 and S1
- Stigmata of disease, e.g. hair-tuft spine base is characteristic of spina bifida occulta.

Feel

- For tenderness, heat and swelling:
  - Paraspinals

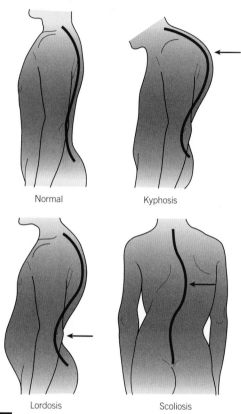

Normal   Kyphosis

Lordosis   Scoliosis

FIGURE 2.16

Possible appearances of posture on inspection. *(Adapted from Ford et al 2005.)*

- Spine (processes):
  - Characteristic step felt in spondylolisthesis.

Move

- Neck/cervical spine (Figure 2.17):
  - Flexion (80°) and extension (60°)
  - Rotation left and right (0–80°)
  - Lateral flexion left and right (0–45°)
- Thoracic spine is almost rigid due to rib cage and sternum
- Lumbar spine (Figure 2.18):
  - Flexion (touch your toes) and extension
  - Rotation left and right of the thoracic spine (with patient sitting)
  - Lateral flexion (slide left arm down left leg and vice versa).

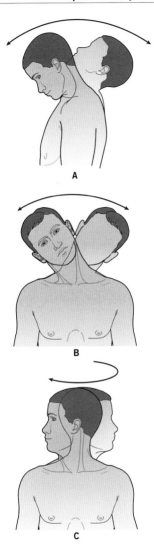

FIGURE 2.17
(**A**) Cervical flexion and extension. (**B**) Cervical lateral flexion. (**C**) Cervical rotation. *(Adapted from Ford et al 2005.)*

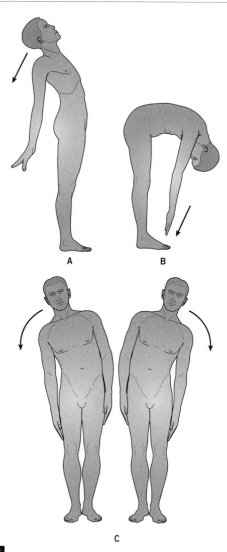

FIGURE 2.18

(**A**) Spine extension. (**B**) Spine flexion. (**C**) Spinal lateral flexion. *(Adapted from Ford et al 2005.)*

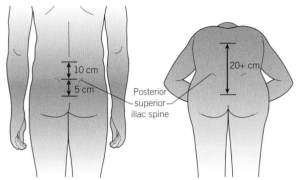

FIGURE 2.19

Schober test. From the midline, two marks are placed 5 cm inferiorly and 10 cm superiorly to the level of the posterior superior iliac spines. During spinal flexion the superior mark should normally displace upwards ≥5 cm. Less than this would be an indication of pathology such as ankylosing spondylitis. *(Adapted from Ford et al 2005.)*

Special Tests

- Schober test (Figure 2.19)
- Sciatica (L4-L5 or L5-S1 disc prolapse):
  - Lasègue straight-leg test: patient is supine with leg fully extended, raise leg from the bed (straight leg raise). Pain and/or paraesthesia present at back of the leg and foot of affected side if positive
  - Braggard test: positive when pain and/or paraesthesia increases on dorsiflexion of the ankle during the straight leg raise
- Femoral nerve irritation (L2-L3 or L3-L4 disc prolapse):
  - With the patient prone and their leg fully extended, raise the leg from the couch (femoral stretch test). Pain and/or paraesthesia present in front of thigh if positive
- Peripheral neurological examination:
  - Remember a complete neurological examination of upper and/or lower limbs is required in the presence of a spinal disorder (Table 2.5, Figure 2.20). Do not neglect to check for saddle anaesthesia and rectal tone in possible cauda equina syndrome.

 HINTS AND TIPS

SPINE

If there is an apparent scoliosis of the spine, remember to ask the patient to bend forward and inspect from behind. Emphasis of the rib hump (thorax convex side) is indicative of idiopathic thoracic scoliosis, but if the deformity is obliterated this is indicative of a flexible curve secondary to another deformity, e.g. leg length inequality. Kyphosis in an elderly individual is strongly suggestive of multiple vertebral fractures especially when there has been >2.5 cm height loss.

TABLE 2.5

THE MYOTOMES, DERMATOMES AND REFLEXES OF THE UPPER AND LOWER LIMBS

Level	Myotome	Dermatome	Reflex
Upper Limb			
C5	Deltoid (shoulder abduction)	Lateral arm	Biceps tendon
C6	Elbow flexion/wrist extension	Lateral forearm	Brachioradialis
C7	Elbow extension/wrist flexion	Middle finger	Triceps
C8	Thumb extension/long finger flexors	Medial forearm	–
T1	Finger abduction (hand interossei)	Medial arm	–
Lower Limb			
L2	Hip flexion	Anterior thigh/groin	–
L3	Knee extension	Anterior and lateral thigh	Patellar tendon
L4	Ankle dorsiflexion	Medial leg and foot	Patellar tendon
L5	Great toe extension (extensor hallucis longus)	Lateral leg and dorsum of foot	–
S1	Ankle plantar flexion	Lateral foot and little toe	Achilles tendon

Reproduced from Table 35.2 in Datta PK, Bulstrode CJK, Nixon IJ. MCQs and EMQs in Surgery: A Bailey & Love Revision Guide. 2nd edition. CRC Press; 2015.

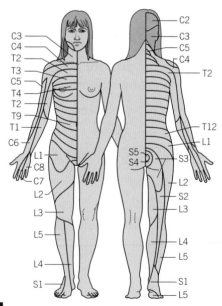

FIGURE 2.20

Dermatome body map.

CHAPTER OUTLINE

ROUTINE HAEMATOLOGY AND BIOCHEMISTRY

Full Blood Count

Abnormalities of the full blood count are common in inflammatory rheumatic diseases (Table 3.1) and full blood count should be performed routinely in the assessment of these patients. It is also customary to perform full blood count prior to orthopaedic surgery in the elderly to exclude anaemia, as well as postoperatively in selected patients. It is important to be vigilant for occult haematological malignancies in both children and adults with an abnormal full blood count.

Coagulation

Coagulation screening is indicated preoperatively for both trauma and elective patients who take warfarin. It should also be performed in patients with a background of bleeding diathesis, haematological disorders (e.g. haemophilia), chronic liver disease (e.g. cirrhosis), sepsis (DIC), and after major haemorrhage. The screen routinely includes the prothrombin time (extrinsic pathway), the activated partial thromboplastin time (intrinsic pathway) and fibrinogen. To standardize the reporting of prothrombin time, the international normalized ratio is also reported. The prothrombin time can be increased secondary to:

- Warfarin
- Liver disease
- DIC.

The APTT can be increased secondary to:

- Unfractionated heparin
- DIC
- Haemophilia A/B.

The D-dimer peptide is a measure of clot formation and is used to exclude the presence of a postoperative venous thromboembolism. However, it has poor specificity because levels rise postoperatively and in patients with infections or inflammatory disease.

TABLE 3.1

THE POTENTIAL CONDITIONS ASSOCIATED WITH ABNORMALITIES OF THE FULL BLOOD COUNT DIFFERENTIAL

Analysis	Condition(s) Indicated
Haemoglobin	
Normochromic normocytic anaemia	Acute/chronic inflammation, malignancy, autoimmune disease
Hypochromic microcytic anaemia	GI bleeding secondary to NSAID, failure of iron utilisation secondary to inflammation
White Cell Count	
Neutrophilia	Bacterial infection/sepsis, steroids, systemic vasculitis
Neutropenia	Felty syndrome, SLE, DMARD therapy
Lymphopenia	SLE, DMARD therapy, viral infection
Eosinophilia	Churg–Strauss syndrome
Platelets	
Thrombocytosis	Acute/chronic inflammation
Thrombocytopenia	DMARD therapy, Felty syndrome, SLE, infection

Erythrocyte Sedimentation Rate and C-Reactive Protein

Measurements of the ESR and CRP are useful in the assessment of patients thought to have inflammatory rheumatic diseases and infections. The CRP is more specific and rises within 10 hours of the onset of infection and inflammation. Elevations in ESR occur more slowly in response to infections and inflammation, and there are other possible causes such as anaemia and multiple myeloma. In these situations the CRP may be normal. Conversely, ESR can be normal in patients with polycythaemia who develop infections and inflammation.

Infections and inflammation can cause other laboratory abnormalities that are collectively termed the acute phase response. This is characterized by:

• Normochromic, normocytic anaemia
• Neutrophilia
• Thrombocytosis
• Raised CRP and ESR
• Reduced albumin level.

Creatinine Kinase

Serum CK is useful in the investigation of muscle disease since levels are elevated as the result of muscle damage. Usually total CK levels are measured although it is possible to measure the CK-MB isoenzyme, which is specific for cardiac muscle, or the CK-MM, which is found in skeletal muscle and smooth muscle. Causes of an elevated CK include:

• Compartment syndrome
• Muscular dystrophy
• Myositis

TABLE 3.2

THE BIOCHEMICAL DERANGEMENTS ASSOCIATED WITH COMMON BONE DISEASE

	Serum Ca²⁺	Serum PO₄³⁻	Serum ALP	Serum PTH	Serum 25(OH)D
Osteoporosis	N	N	N	N	N/↓
Paget disease	N	N	↑↑	N	N/↓
Osteomalacia	N/↓	↓	↑	↑	↓↓
Renal osteodystrophy	↓	↑↑	↑	↑↑	N/↓
Primary hyperparathyroidism	↑	N/↓	N/↑	↑	N/↓

↑: increased; ↓: decreased; N: within normal range.

- Alcohol, drugs, excessive exercise, trauma, postoperatively
- African-Caribbean origin (levels are normally higher than those for Caucasians).

Patients suspected to have myositis or myopathies usually require additional tests, such as electromyography or needle muscle biopsy, to confirm the diagnosis (discussed later).

Routine Biochemistry

Routine biochemistry (U&E, LFT, calcium, phosphate, albumin) is useful in the assessment of patients with inflammatory rheumatic diseases, bone diseases and malignancy. Urea and electrolytes are routinely assessed in the perioperative period after major orthopaedic surgery.

Some bone diseases are associated with characteristic alterations in serum calcium, phosphate and alkaline phosphatase as summarized in Table 3.2. Raised uric acid levels predispose to gout but values can be elevated in obesity and metabolic syndrome in patients who may never develop gout. Conversely, uric acid levels may be normal during an acute attack of gout since levels decrease during acute inflammation. Abnormalities of renal function may also occur in patients with rheumatic diseases, and may occur as the result of renal involvement in SLE, connective tissue disorders, vasculitis and gout or as the result of treatment with nephrotoxic agents such as cyclosporine and NSAIDs. Abnormalities of LFT (particularly ALP) are common during flares of inflammatory rheumatic disease as the result of inflammation. Another common cause of abnormal LFTs is hepatotoxicity due to methotrexate and other DMARDs.

 HINTS AND TIPS

ROUTINE HAEMATOLOGY AND BIOCHEMISTRY

Elevations in CRP and ESR can occur postoperatively in the absence of infection with a peak at 48 to 72 hours and returning to normal within 3 weeks of surgery. Raised uric acid levels are typical in patients with a history of gout except during an acute attack when levels may be normal. Normochromic normocytic anaemia is common in patients with inflammatory rheumatic diseases.

IMMUNOLOGY

Anti-Citrullinated Peptide Antibodies

Testing for anti-citrullinated peptide antibodies (ACPA) is useful in the assessment of patients with inflammatory arthritis. Raised levels of antibodies are present in about 70% of patients with RA (which is termed 'seropositive' RA) but are negative in the remaining 30% (seronegative RA). The ACPA have higher specificity (>95%) for the diagnosis of RA than RF, although positive results can be obtained in some diseases like autoimmune hepatitis. It is of interest that ACPA can be present for months or years before the disease presents clinically. Patients who are ACPA positive have a worse prognosis and more severe disease than those who are ACPA negative, and patients with rheumatoid nodules are almost always ACPA positive. The majority of patients who are ACPA positive are also RF positive.

Rheumatoid Factor

Testing for rheumatoid factor (RF) may be performed in the assessment of patients with inflammatory arthritis but has been largely superseded by ACPA. About 60–70% of patients with RA are RF positive, but false positives are found in many other situations including CTD, SLE, chronic infections, chronic liver disease and malignancy. The test may also be positive in some healthy elderly individuals. Patients with rheumatoid nodules are almost always RF positive. Patients who are RF positive have more severe disease and a poorer prognosis than RF-negative individuals.

Anti-Nuclear Antibody

Testing for anti-nuclear antibodies (ANA) is useful in the assessment of patients suspected of having SLE or CTD. The test involves adding a sample of the patient serum to a cultured cell line in vitro and looking for evidence of antibody binding to the nucleus using indirect immunofluorescence microscopy. The results are usually reported in terms of the titre of serum at which the test becomes positive (e.g. 1 in 80, 1 in 160, etc.). The higher the titre, the greater the clinical significance. Causes of a positive ANA include:

- SLE
- Systemic sclerosis
- Connective tissue disease
- Sjögren syndrome
- RA.

A weakly positive ANA can also be found in normal individuals and patients with:

- Autoimmune disease, chronic hepatitis, thyroid disorders
- Myasthenia gravis
- Widespread burns.

A positive ANA test is supportive of the diagnosis of SLE and CTD when found in the presence of other clinical features but cannot be used on its own to make the diagnosis.

Anti-Double Stranded DNA Antibodies

Anti-double stranded DNA (dsDNA) antibodies are highly specific for the diagnosis of SLE. They are indicated to confirm the diagnosis of SLE in patients with suggestive clinical features who test positive for ANA. Patients with drug-induced lupus are typically negative for dsDNA antibodies.

Antibodies to Nuclear Antigens

Testing for antibodies to extractable nuclear antigens is useful in the assessment of patients with CTD, SLE and inflammatory myositis. The presence of certain antibodies is associated with some clinical features but the specificity and sensitivity of individual tests is poor. Known associations include:

- Anti-La – SLE, Sjögren syndrome
- Anti-Jo-1 – polymyositis
- Anti-Scl-70 – scleroderma
- Anti-centromere antibodies – mixed CTD
- Anti-Sm antibodies – SLE and renal involvement
- Anti-Ro antibodies – SLE. Associated with neonatal SLE and foetal heart block.

Anti-Neutrophil Cytoplasmic Antibodies

Measurement of anti neutrophil cytoplasmic antibodies (ANCA) is useful for the assessment of patients suspected to have vasculitis. These antibodies recognize enzymes present within the neutrophil cytoplasm. There are two main subtypes:

1. Anti-PR3-ANCA (cytoplasmic): these recognize the enzyme proteinase-3 and are associated with granulomatosis with polyangiitis (also known as Wegener granulomatosis).
2. Anti-MPO-ANCA (perinuclear): these antibodies target the enzyme myeloperoxidase and are associated with other microscopic angiitis and Churg–Strauss vasculitis.

The tests are not completely specific because a positive MPO-ANCA can also be found in patients with inflammatory bowel disease or a neoplasm.

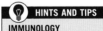 **HINTS AND TIPS**

IMMUNOLOGY

Testing for autoantibodies is useful in helping to confirm the correct diagnosis in patients with clinical features suggestive of autoimmune disease. The presence of a positive antibody test in isolation is seldom significant.

JOINT ASPIRATION AND SYNOVIAL FLUID ANALYSIS

This is a key investigation in patients with an acute swollen joint. It can be used for diagnostic and therapeutic aspiration/injection in:

- Acute monoarthritis to establish diagnosis, in particular sepsis
- Order to relieve capsular tension in acute haemarthrosis

TABLE 3.3

CHARACTERISTICS OF INFLAMMATORY AND NONINFLAMMATORY SYNOVIAL FLUID*

	Noninflammatory Synovial Aspirate	Inflammatory Synovial Aspirate
Volume	Small	Large
Cell Number	Low	High (leading to turbidity)
Appearance	Clear and colourless/pale yellow	Cloudy, translucent or opaque fluid with pus (pyarthrosis related to neutrophilia) and/or blood staining (haemarthrosis)
Viscosity	High due to hyaluronate	Low due to breakdown of hyaluronate

*A deposit of lipid floating on a haemarthrosis is indicative of an intraarticular fracture.

- Local anaesthetic +/− steroid to localize the anatomical source of pain, (e.g. rotator cuff impingement)
- Steroid injection to manage degenerative or inflammatory arthropathy
- Local or regional nerve blockade prior to fracture/dislocation manipulation.

In patients with inflammatory arthritis, leukocytes are increased in number, the fluid is cloudy and viscosity is reduced. As the severity of joint inflammation increases (OA < RA < seronegative arthritis < crystal arthritis < septic arthritis), the synovial fluid takes on the characteristics shown in Table 3.3. Analysis of synovial fluid can provide diagnostic information in the following conditions:

- Acute gout – inflammatory infiltrate and urate crystals
- Pseudogout – inflammatory infiltrate and calcium pyrophosphate crystals
- Reactive arthritis – inflammatory infiltrate
- Intraarticular bleeding – blood or blood stained fluid
- Trauma with an associated effusion – blood or blood stained fluid
- Septic arthritis – inflammatory infiltrate and positive culture.

Relative contraindications/cautions are:

- Risk of inducing septic arthritis (e.g. systemic infection, overlying cellulitis)
- Coagulation defect (e.g. bleeding disorder, anticoagulants)
- Prosthetic joint
- Allergy to intended drug or constituents.

Potential complications are:

- Infection
- Bleeding
- Transient worsening of symptoms for 24–48 hours (steroid flare).

It is customary to send synovial fluid to microbiology even though sepsis might not be suspected. If sepsis is suspected the sample should be marked urgent and antibiotic sensitivities requested. The most common organism in septic arthritis is *Staphylococcus aureus*. This and other organisms, commonly sourced from the patient's skin or blood, are often implicated in infection of prosthetic joints or implants. Less common organisms are streptococci, TB and gonococcus.

Polarized light microscopy is especially useful in the diagnosis of gout and pseudogout. In gout, long needle-shaped sodium urate crystals may be identified with strong light intensity and negative birefringence. In pseudogout: small rhomboid or rod-shaped calcium pyrophosphate crystals may be seen. These are fewer in number, with weak birefringence.

 PROCEDURE

JOINT ASPIRATION

CONSENT

- Low risk of introducing sepsis
- Cartilage/tendon damage with multiple injections
- Transient worsening of symptoms after injection
- Skin hypopigmentation and lipodystrophy (skin dimpling)

PROCEDURE

'Clean' location, aseptic technique and ensuring the following materials are to hand:

- Dressing pack, sterile gloves, syringe and hypodermic needles
- Skin preparation and local anaesthetic
- Sterile collecting container if aspiration planned
- Nature of aspirate documented, e.g. straw/turbid/purulent/blood/haemoserous

KNEE

Infiltrate the skin and soft tissue with local anaesthetic and advance the needle until the joint cavity is reached. For aspiration a medial or lateral soft point 1 cm medial or lateral to the border of the patella with the knee in full extension is used. Palpate the soft spot between the patella border, the anterior aspect of the femoral condyle and the tibial plateau.

For injection a medial parapatellar tendon approach can be used. Place the knee in 90° of flexion and identify the soft spot within a triangle bordered by the patellar tendon, the medial tibial plateau and the medial femoral condyle.

SHOULDER

The subacromial bursa is approached posteriorly immediately under the inferior edge of the palpable acromion process, aiming anteriorly and 15° superiorly. The glenohumeral joint is approached posteriorly. Identify the glenohumeral articulation by firm palpation with the thumb as a soft spot 3 cm below the acromion process. Identify the coracoid process anteriorly with the tip of the index finger. Mark both points. The needle passes along a line between the two points.

 HINTS AND TIPS

JOINT ASPIRATION AND SYNOVIAL FLUID ANALYSIS

Synovial fluid should be sent for urgent microscopy when septic arthritis is suspected. The absence of organisms does not rule out infection, particularly if the patient has already received antibiotic therapy.

IMAGING

Radiographs

Plain radiographs (X-rays) remain an essential diagnostic tool within rheumatology and orthopaedics. The following should be looked for:

- General: name, age, date of film, view, part of body and adequacy of film
- Soft tissues: wasting, swelling, calcification and free air
- Bones: fracture and classification (see Chapter 4), deformity, cysts, calcification, osteopenia or osteosclerosis
- Joints: joint space, erosions, calcification, sclerosis and new bone formation.

The Ottawa Ankle Rules state radiographs are indicated if there are any of the following:

- Inability to weight-bear immediately and/or four steps in the emergency department
- Bony tenderness along the distal 6 cm of the posterior edge or tip of the medial malleolus
- Bony tenderness along the distal 6 cm of the posterior edge or tip of the lateral malleolus
- Bony tenderness at the base of the navicular or fifth metatarsal bone in foot injuries, which require a foot radiograph.

The Ottawa Knee Rules state radiographs are required if there are any of the following:

- Age 55 or over
- Inability to weight bear immediately and/or four steps in the emergency department
- Inability to flex the knee to 90°
- Bony tenderness over the fibula head
- Isolated bony tenderness of the patella.

For details on interpreting children's radiographs, see Chapter 7.

Dual Energy X-Ray Absorptiometry

Dual energy X-ray absorptiometry (DEXA) is indicated in patients suspected to have osteoporosis. It should be considered in patients with low trauma fractures above the age of 50, patients suspected to have vertebral fractures and patients with risk factors for osteoporosis in whom fracture risk assessment using QFracture® or FRAX® tools have yielded a 10-year fracture risk of >10%. Repeat DEXA scans at intervals of not less than 2 years can be used to monitor the response to treatment or progression of osteopenia. The principle of DEXA is shown in Figure 3.1. Scans are usually performed at hip and spine. The most important result to look at is the T-score which represents the number of standard deviations by which the BMD deviates from the population average for healthy individuals with peak bone mass. Osteoporosis is diagnosed when the T-score is <−2.5 at the spine or hip (Table 3.4). The Z-score represents the number of standard deviations by which the value deviates from the population

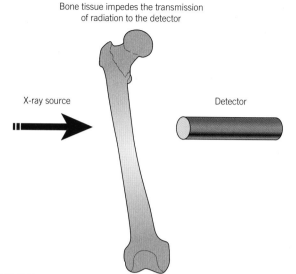

Bone tissue impedes the transmission
of radiation to the detector

X-ray source

Detector

FIGURE 3.1

The principle of DEXA scanning. The BMD is calculated by determining the
reduction in expected radiation, which is related to the amount of bone mineral
available to absorb the radiation. This is converted into a measurement of BMD in
grams of hydroxyapatite/cm^2 by calibrating against an internal standard.

TABLE 3.4

DEFINITIONS BASED ON DEXA SCANNING RESULTS

T-Score	WHO* Diagnosis
Greater than −1	Normal
−1.0 → −2.5	Osteopenia
Below −2.5	Osteoporosis

*World Health Organisation. These categories only apply to postmenopausal women and men above the age of 50 years.

average in age-matched controls. The Z-score should be used in preference to
the T-score in children. Since osteoporosis increases in prevalence with age it is
important to remember that elderly people often have osteoporosis (T-score of
−2.5) in the presence of a normal Z-score.

Ultrasound

Ultrasound is a useful procedure for:

• Assessment of periarticular structures, e.g. popliteal cyst, patellar tendon,
Achilles tendon and shoulder rotator cuff

- Assessment of soft tissues and joint fluid, e.g. a hip joint effusion in transient synovitis of the hip
- Assessment of subclinical synovitis in patients suspected to have inflammatory arthritis
- Assessment for postoperative deep vein thrombosis
- Joint aspiration and injection (particularly for inaccessible joints such as the hip)
- Real-time guidance for needle biopsy.

Bone Scintigraphy

This is a useful technique in the assessment of patients suspected of having bone tumours or metastases and Paget disease of bone. It involves injection of ^{99m}Tc-bisphosphonate followed by skeletal imaging with a gamma camera. Increased uptake of the radionuclide early after the injection reflects blood flow and increased uptake later reflects increased bone remodelling. Although increases in isotope uptake are nonspecific, the patterns of increase in different disorders are often quite characteristic allowing a diagnosis to be made.

Computerized Tomography

Computerised tomography (CT) allows 3D imaging of complex intraarticular fractures (Figure 3.2), the spinal canal and facet joints, as well as showing alterations in skeletal anatomy. It is rapid and not subject to 'movement artifact'.

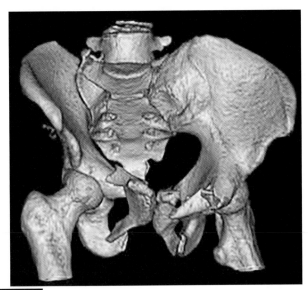

FIGURE 3.2
A 3D-CT reconstruction of a pelvic fracture.

It is also used for staging for both primary and secondary bone tumours. There are, however, limitations due to a large radiation exposure and inadequate visualization of soft tissues. Single photon emission computed tomography (SPECT) involves a combination of CT scan imaging and radionuclide imaging with a gamma camera following an injection of radiopharmaceutical. It is useful in the assessment of bone metastases, Paget disease and primary hyperparathyroidism.

Magnetic Resonance Imaging

Magnetic resonance imaging (MRI) gives highly detailed information on skeletal anatomy, soft tissues and intraarticular structures such as cartilage. Gadolinium enhancement may be useful in the assessment of inflammatory conditions. Common applications of MRI are in the assessment of:

- Spinal disease (disc prolapse, nerve root or cord compression)
- Axial spondyloarthropathy
- Osteonecrosis (e.g. Perthes disease)
- Soft tissue, bone and joint infection or tumour
- Chronic regional pain syndrome (CRPS)
- Subclinical synovitis
- Meniscal and rotator cuff tears, ligament injuries (Figure 3.3).

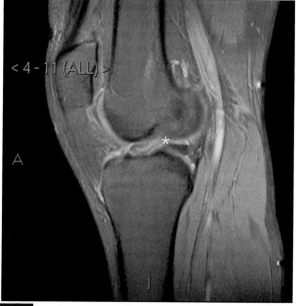

FIGURE 3.3

An MRI sagittal view demonstrating a rupture of the anterior cruciate ligament (ACL).

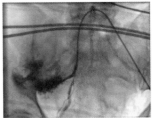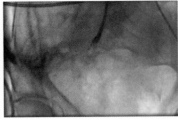

Interventional angiography performed with embolization following a complex pelvis fracture.

Angiography

Angiography is of value in the assessment of patients suspected of having medium or large vessel vasculitis. It involves the injection of contrast medium into the vascular system followed by imaging with MRI or CT. It can frequently provide diagnostic information in polyarteritis nodosa, cerebral vasculitis and Takayasu disease. It can also be used to assess for postoperative pulmonary embolus (CTPA – CT pulmonary angiography) and vascular injuries associated with a fracture, including interventional embolization for unstable patients with a pelvic fracture (Figure 3.4).

> ### 💡 HINTS AND TIPS
>
> **IMAGING**
>
> Radiographs are the imaging method of choice for the investigation of fractures. For limb fractures quality radiographs should include the joint above and below. MRI is especially helpful in spinal disease and to investigate complex soft tissue injuries, particularly around the knee.

TISSUE BIOPSY

Tissue biopsy can give useful diagnostic information value in many inflammatory conditions most notably vasculitis and SLE, as well as being essential to the diagnosis of bone and soft tissue masses. The aim of a biopsy is to provide a representative tissue sample of the area in question and is indicated when noninvasive investigations have failed to provide a definitive diagnosis. Soft tissue or bone lesions often require a biopsy to confirm the diagnosis. It is routinely performed once advanced imaging has been performed. Increasingly, biopsies are performed by radiologists under imaging control. Close cooperation between surgeon, radiologist and pathologist is vital. Types of biopsy include fine needle aspiration, core biopsy, incisional biopsy and excisional biopsy. Applications include:

- Muscle biopsy: inflammatory myositis or myopathy
- Renal biopsy or skin biopsy: small vessel vasculitis, SLE, polyangiitis with granulomatosis

- Biopsy of nasal passages or lung biopsy: polyangiitis with granulomatosis
- Bone and/or soft tissue biopsy: osteomalacia, infection, Paget disease, infiltrative disorders, primary or secondary bone or soft tissue tumours.

 HINTS AND TIPS

TISSUE BIOPSY

Biopsy when tumour is expected should ideally be carried out by a recognized musculoskeletal tumour service. Key principles of a safe open biopsy include use of a longitudinal incision that can be incorporated in the excision during definitive surgery, violation of the affected compartment only, meticulous haemostasis and avoidance of neurovascular structures.

ARTHROSCOPY

Arthroscopy is frequently used in both the diagnosis and repair of soft tissue problems within the joint, commonly of the shoulder or knee. It is less commonly performed in the wrist, elbow, hip and ankle. It can be used in the acute washout of septic joints. Potential complications include bleeding, neurovascular injury, damage to the joint or infection.

 PROCEDURE

KNEE ARTHROSCOPY

INDICATIONS

- Diagnostic
- Therapeutic:
  - Debridement or repair of meniscal tears
  - Cruciate ligament reconstruction
  - Chondral defect procedures
  - Synovectomy
  - Washout for sepsis
  - Lateral release
  - Removal of loose body.

CONSENT

- Bleeding
- Infection
- Neurovascular damage.

PROCEDURE

The patient may be positioned in a variety of manners for knee arthroscopy. In principle, varus and valgus stress needs to be placed on the knee to open the medial and lateral compartments to provide access. This is delivered by placing the femur in a clamp, or by a post attached to the side of the table. A tourniquet is routinely used.

Accurate placement of the portals is essential for access of the camera and instruments. These are placed either side of the patellar tendon, just below the patella, in an oblique manner. Care should be taken not to damage the menisci by aiming too low. The lateral portal is routinely made first. The portal is created with a small incision followed by a blunt inner trocar passed into the lateral

Continued

PROCEDURE—cont'd

compartment of the knee and is initially introduced with the knee flexed, aiming towards the intercondylar notch. The knee is then carefully extended and the trocar is advanced into the patellofemoral compartment. The camera is white balanced and then inserted with areas of the knee inspected in turn. This will include the patellofemoral compartment, medial and lateral compartments and gutters, and the intercondylar notch.

The medial portal is then made under direct vision of the camera and can be used as a passage for instruments. Further portals are possible, e.g. suprapatellar, and the camera can be moved to the medial portal with instruments passed through the lateral portal if so required. Once the procedure is complete, the portal wounds can be closed with sterile adhesive or nylon sutures.

Chapter 4

Trauma, Injury Classification and Perioperative Care

CHAPTER OUTLINE

TRAUMA ASSESSMENT	PREOPERATIVE MANAGEMENT
INJURY ASSESSMENT, CLASSIFICATION AND MANAGEMENT	POSTOPERATIVE MANAGEMENT
	FRACTURE COMPLICATIONS

TRAUMA ASSESSMENT

Initial assessment and resuscitation of the trauma patient should follow advanced trauma life support (ATLS) guidelines:

- Primary survey (ABCDE):
  - **A**irway with C-spine control
  - **B**reathing and ventilation
  - **C**irculation with shock control:
    - Shock is defined as an acute circulatory failure resulting in inadequate tissue perfusion, anaerobic metabolism and subsequent end organ injury
    - Classification of hypovolaemic shock (Table 4.1)
    - Causes of shock include hypovolaemic, cardiogenic, septic, neurogenic and anaphylactic
    - Hypovolaemic shock is most commonly seen in trauma patients, and the five places blood can be found include the chest, abdomen, pelvis, long bones and the floor/scene
  - **D**isability
  - **E**xposure and environment
- Secondary survey (when primary survey complete): including full body examination, a neurological examination where possible and appropriate further imaging (e.g. CT). The character and degree of the patient's injuries should now have been assessed.

Within this, life-threatening injuries should be dealt with immediately. Monitor vitals at all times (pulse, BP, oxygen saturation, respiratory rate, Glasgow Coma Scale (GCS), blood glucose, urine output); wide bore venous access, full blood count, clinical biochemistry and arterial blood gas (ABG) analysis are routine. Oxygen and fluid resuscitation (e.g. crystalloid, blood) are the mainstays of treatment, with additional immediate management of life-threatening injuries. Adjunctive imaging of the primary survey includes chest, C-spine and pelvic radiographs. Once the patient's condition has been stabilized, further injury assessment and management can begin (Figure 4.1).

TABLE 4.1

CLASSIFICATION OF HYPOVOLAEMIC SHOCK (ADVANCED TRAUMA AND LIFE SUPPORT MANUAL)

Class of Shock	1	2	3	4
Blood loss (mL)	<750	750–1500	1500–2000	2000+
% of blood volume (70-kg adult)	15	15–30	30–40	40+
Pulse rate	<100	>100	>120	140+
Blood pressure	↔	↔	↓	↓
Pulse pressure	↔	↓	↓	↓
Respiratory rate (breaths/min)	14–20	20–30	30–40	>40
Urine output (mL/h)	>30	20–30	5–15	Negligible
CNS status	Restless	Anxious	Anxious and confused	Confused and lethargic

 HINTS AND TIPS

OVERVIEW OF TRAUMA ASSESSMENT

Follow the ATLS guidelines. **AMPLE** is the mnemonic used to efficiently gain important details regarding an injury and includes **a**llergies, **m**edication and tetanus, **p**ast medical history, **l**ast meal and **e**vents of the incident. A patient who is talking by definition has a patent airway, but this can become compromised and reassessment is a cornerstone of ATLS protocol. A GCS of less than or equal to eight is an indication for anaesthetic involvement to attain a definitive airway. In the multiply injured patient, a thorough and complete secondary survey is essential to exclude any further injuries once initial lifesaving assessment and management has been achieved. Early CT of head, chest, abdomen and pelvis is becoming more popular, but the patient must be in a stable condition for this to occur safely. Normal cervical spine CT imaging does not allow definitive clearance, especially in children, and repeated clinical assessment with MRI may be indicated.

INJURY ASSESSMENT, CLASSIFICATION AND MANAGEMENT

Initial Injury Assessment

History

During the initial assessment of a suspected fracture or soft tissue injury it is important to determine the history and mechanism of the injury (see Chapter 2), including the likely cause:

- Trauma causes damage to normal bone and/or soft tissue due to a direct or, more commonly, indirect force. It is useful to classify this in terms of the causative force, e.g. low energy *vs.* high energy, blunt *vs.* penetrating, crush, and multiple (major) trauma.
- Pathological, where the injury or fracture occurs in an already compromised, abnormally weak structure, e.g. a pathological fracture due to a bone cyst or bony metastasis.

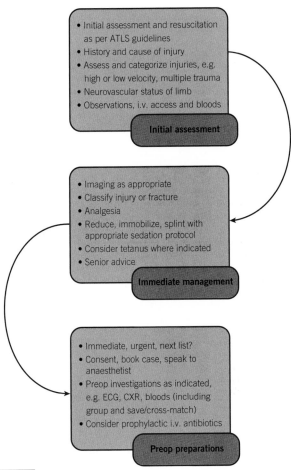

- Initial assessment and resuscitation as per ATLS guidelines
- History and cause of injury
- Assess and categorize injuries, e.g. high or low velocity, multiple trauma
- Neurovascular status of limb
- Observations, i.v. access and bloods

Initial assessment

- Imaging as appropriate
- Classify injury or fracture
- Analgesia
- Reduce, immobilize, splint with appropriate sedation protocol
- Consider tetanus where indicated
- Senior advice

Immediate management

- Immediate, urgent, next list?
- Consent, book case, speak to anaesthetist
- Preop investigations as indicated, e.g. ECG, CXR, bloods (including group and save/cross-match)
- Consider prophylactic i.v. antibiotics

Preop preparations

FIGURE 4.1

An overview of injury assessment. Local anaesthetic may be required to complete a thorough assessment, e.g. a digital nerve block for a finger. Any neurovascular deficit needs to be determined prior to this.

- Stress or fatigue, where repeated stress on the bone leads to injury, e.g. second metatarsal neck fractures in army recruits ('march fracture').

For all injuries, but particularly upper limb injuries, it is useful to determine the occupation and handedness of the patient. In addition, it is useful to ascertain from the patient what function they have lost as a result of their injury, as well as how this might have changed/worsened since the time of injury.

Examination (see Chapter 2)

Examine the affected and surrounding joint(s) and soft tissue for:

- Pain, bruising and tenderness
- Swelling, redness, heat or crepitus
- Range of movement (active and passive)
- Gross deformity, e.g. secondary to rotation, shortening or possible dislocation (a comparison with the unaffected limb can be helpful)
- Foreign bodies in wounds and potential soft tissue damage, e.g. nerves or tendons in open hand injuries
- Loss of function, power or sensation.

Neurovascular Status

Assessment of the neurovascular status of the limb(s) is critical, and neglect at this stage can lead to avoidable complications (see Chapters 1 and 2). This includes examination of pulses, capillary refill time, colour and sensation distal to the injury site. Doppler may be used as part of the vascular assessment. Some key examples of susceptible soft tissue injuries are as follows.

NERVES

- Axillary: following a shoulder (anterior) dislocation and subsequent reduction, ± a proximal humeral fracture
- Radial: following a mid/distal shaft humeral or supracondylar fracture, elbow fracture/dislocation
- Posterior interosseous: following a Monteggia fracture-dislocation or isolated radial head or neck injury
- Anterior interosseous: following a supracondylar fracture of the humerus
- Median: wrist laceration or fracture-dislocation
- Ulnar: following a supracondylar fracture of the humerus, elbow fracture-dislocation in adults, wrist laceration
- Digital: following a laceration to the fingers or thumb (sensation and sweating are key features for testing)
- Sciatic: following a posterior hip dislocation or acetabular fracture
- Femoral: following a pubic ramus fracture (rare)
- Tibial: following a knee dislocation or tibial fracture
- Common peroneal: following a fibular neck fracture or knee dislocation.

BLOOD VESSELS (DIVISION, COMPRESSION, STRETCHING, SPASM)

- Axillary artery: following a shoulder dislocation
- Brachial artery: in supracondylar fractures of the humerus or following an elbow dislocation
- Radial artery: following a wrist laceration
- Ulnar artery: following a wrist laceration
- Digital artery: following a laceration to the fingers or thumb (if the artery is damaged it is probable that the nerve is damaged also)
- Deep femoral artery (profunda femoris): following a fracture of the femur
- Lumbosacral plexus, iliac vessels or superior gluteal artery: following a pelvic fracture
- Popliteal artery: following a knee dislocation or proximal tibial fracture.

TABLE 4.2		
FINGER AND THUMB FLEXOR TENDON INJURY ZONES		
Zone	**From**	**To**
Finger		
1	Midpoint middle phalanx	Finger tip
2	Distal palmar crease (A1 pulley)	Midpoint middle phalanx
3	Distal edge carpal tunnel	Distal palmar crease (A1 pulley)
4	Proximal edge carpal tunnel	Distal edge carpal tunnel
5	Forearm and wrist	Proximal edge carpal tunnel
Thumb		
1	IPJ	Finger tip
2	A1 pulley (proximal phalanx)	IPJ
3	Thenar muscles	Distal palmar crease
4	Proximal edge carpal tunnel	Distal edge carpal tunnel
5	Musculotendinous junction	Proximal edge carpal tunnel

Adapted from Tables 55.1 and 55.2 in Datta PK, Bulstrode CJK, Wallace WFM. MRCS Part A: 500 SBAs and EMQs. 1st edition. JP Medical Publishers; 2012.

MUSCLES AND TENDONS (SPRAIN, RUPTURE, DIVISION, CRUSH AND ISCHAEMIA)

- Long flexors and extensors to fingers (e.g. flexor digitorum superficialis and flexor digitorum profundus): following a wrist, hand or finger laceration:
  - Verden zones for flexor tendon injury (Table 4.2, Figure 4.2)
- Thumb flexors: following a wrist or thumb laceration (Table 4.2, Figure 4.2)
- Tendon sheath: direct contamination in palm or digital penetrating injury leading to infection (Figure 4.2):
  - Kanavel's signs for a flexor tendon sheath infection:
    - Finger held in flexion
    - Fusiform swelling of the tendon and digit
    - Tenderness on palpation over the tendon sheath
    - Pain on passive extension of the affected digit
- EPL tendon: delayed rupture may occur after a distal radius fracture.

Imaging

Consider the appropriate imaging required at this point:

- Dependent on suspected injury and area(s) of body affected
- Radiographs can also be helpful to determine foreign body invasion of soft tissues:
  - Refer to local guidelines for appropriate indications
  - Special reference should be made to the Ottawa Knee and Ankle Rules (see Chapter 3), which provide indications for imaging the knee and ankle, respectively
- Further imaging as indicated:
  - Ultrasound for soft tissue injuries, e.g. rotator cuff
  - CT for spinal, pelvic and complex periarticular fractures
  - MRI for complex soft tissue injuries and spinal injuries.

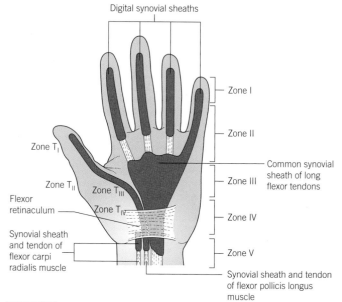

Digital synovial sheaths

Zone I

Zone II

Zone T₍I₎

Zone T₍II₎   Zone T₍III₎

Flexor
retinaculum   Zone T₍IV₎

Synovial sheath
and tendon of
flexor carpi
radialis muscle

Common synovial
sheath of long
flexor tendons

Zone III

Zone IV

Zone V

Synovial sheath and tendon
of flexor pollicis longus
muscle

FIGURE 4.2

Penetrating injuries to the synovial sheaths of the hand can lead to infection
spreading throughout the hand and proximally up the arm. Verdan zones are used
in assessing the location, consequence and treatment of flexor tendon injuries.

Classification of Injury

Classification of Fractures

The classification of individual adult fractures is discussed in Chapter 6 and the
classification of paediatric injuries is discussed in Chapter 7.

Classification of fractures by relation to surrounding tissue:

- Simple or closed: fractures where the overlying skin is intact and the
  fracture site is not communicating with the skin or a body cavity.
- Compound or open: fractures where there is significant soft tissue damage
  leading to broken ends communicating with the skin or body cavity. The
  bone ends may not be seen at presentation (out–in type injury). These are
  prone to infection and subsequent complications. They are classified
  according to Gustilo classification of open fractures (Table 4.3).
- Intraarticular: the fracture involves the joint/articulating surface, e.g. tibial
  plateau fracture.

Classification of fractures by radiographs (Figure 4.3):

- Transverse: caused by a direct blow, with the shape of the fractured bones
  allowing for better fracture alignment and union

TABLE 4.3

GUSTILO CLASSIFICATION OF OPEN FRACTURES

Certain injuries are classified as a grade 3 irrespective of wound size or soft tissue injury, e.g. traumatic amputation, segmental fracture, heavy contamination

Grade	Description
1	Wound less than 1 cm, low energy, clean, no periosteal stripping, minimal soft tissue damage
2	Wound greater than 1 cm, moderate soft tissue damage, no periosteal stripping/flaps/avulsions
3A	Often high-energy, extensive soft tissue damage (e.g. skin, muscle), periosteal stripping, contamination Adequate coverage postfracture stabilization – no flap required
3B	Often high-energy, extensive soft tissue damage (e.g. skin, muscle), periosteal stripping, contamination Inadequate coverage postfracture stabilization – flap required
3C	Open fracture associated with an arterial injury requiring repair

Reproduced from Table 29.1 in Datta PK, Bulstrode CJK, Nixon IJ. MCQs and EMQs in Surgery: A Bailey & Love Revision Guide. 2nd edition. CRC Press; 2015.

- Spiral or oblique: are due to an indirect blow, e.g. twisting, and are unstable and difficult to align
  - Sharp detached fragment of a transverse, spiral or oblique fracture ('butterfly fragment')
- Comminuted/multifragmented/complex: either due to severe direct trauma to the bone or osteoporotic bone, a fracture of ≥2 parts
- Compression/crush: a fracture secondary to compression force, often in pathological bone, e.g. an osteoporotic vertebral crush fracture
- Avulsion: a fracture fragment, often secondary to a ligament or tendon being avulsed off bone, e.g. base of fifth metatarsal fracture
- Descriptive characteristics:
  - Displacement
  - Rotation
  - Angulation
  - Shortening.

Classification of Dislocations

By convention the direction of a dislocation, or fracture-dislocation, is determined by the position of the distal part relative to the proximal:

- Subluxation: when there is some, but not complete, loss of contact between articular surfaces of the joint. This type of injury may need active management to restore normal function.
- Dislocation: when there is absolutely no contact between articular surfaces of the joint, e.g. anterior dislocation of the shoulder. Active treatment is needed.
- Fracture-dislocation: when there is absolutely no contact between articular surfaces of the joint, as with an associated periarticular fracture. Early management is more difficult in this situation, with open reduction and

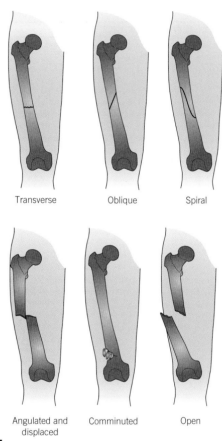

Transverse   Oblique   Spiral

Angulated and displaced   Comminuted   Open

FIGURE 4.3

Fracture classification by pattern and deformity.

internal fixation of fracture fragments +/− ligaments potentially needed, e.g. terrible triad fracture dislocation of the elbow. Fragments can become incarcerated into the joint and block reduction – open reduction and removal of fragment required.

Immediate Injury Management

See individual injury for the recommended management (Chapter 6).

- Initial assessment and resuscitation should follow ATLS guidelines
- Analgesia (see Chapter 8)

TABLE 4.4	
BLOOD LOSS FROM DIFFERENT FRACTURE SITES	
Fracture Site	**Blood Loss (L)**
Pelvic ring, proximal femur	1.5–3
Femur to knee, humerus to elbow	1–2.5
Tibia to ankle, elbow to wrist	0.5–1.5

Adapted from Dandy DJ, Edwards DJ. Essential Orthopaedics and Trauma, 4th edition. Elsevier: Churchill Livingstone; 2003.

- Wound management: an actively bleeding wound should be treated initially with direct pressure on the site and tourniquet as required
- Fractures and dislocations:
  - Fluid resuscitation as blood loss, even in closed fractures, may be large (Table 4.4)
  - Open fractures will require clear documentation/photograph (patient consent, refer to local guidelines), followed by covering with an iodine/saline soaked gauze and sterile dressing:
    - Urgent exploration, washout and debridement, timing is open to debate
    - Extend wound edges, debride all contaminated or devitalized tissue, deliver fracture ends, copious lavage with up to 10 litres of saline
    - Temporary or definitive fracture stabilization
    - Wound left open (unless grade 1), with a return to theatre for further assessment usually within 48 hours
  - Immediate realignment and temporary stabilization of fractures using inline traction with immobilization in the anatomical position, will relieve pain and reduce the risk of (further) soft tissue injury and/or bleeding:
    - Urgent in the presence of skin compromise or neurovascular injury
  - Closed reduction is used to realign the bones to their anatomical position (this is done with appropriate analgesia and sedation); open reduction in theatre may be necessary:
    - Remember to reassess neurovascular status pre- and postreduction
  - Immobilization and/or traction for maintenance of position are achieved by back slab using plaster (e.g. plaster of Paris) or traction (e.g. Thomas splint)
  - Definitive operative stabilization may include internal fixation (wires, plates, screws, intramedullary nails) or external fixation (e.g. Ilizarov ring fixator, or monoaxial frame) of the fracture
- Tetanus and antibiotic prophylaxis should be given for open injuries (refer to local guidelines).

 HINTS AND TIPS

INJURY ASSESSMENT, CLASSIFICATION AND TREATMENT

It is essential to both assess and image the joint above and below for occult injuries, e.g. radial head dislocation associated with a fracture of the ulna shaft. An open fracture associated with farmyard injuries/contaminated wounds is classified as Gustilo grade 3, irrespective of the size of the wound or soft tissue cover. Any fracture associated with an arterial injury requiring repair is automatically a Gustilo grade 3C.

PREOPERATIVE MANAGEMENT

Assessment

Whether elective or emergency surgery is to be carried out, it is important to undertake a thorough assessment before the operation. This should include:

- History and examination (see Chapter 2)
- Co-morbidities:
  - Establish the current health of the patient and baseline level of function
  - Determine the current control of any other medical problems, e.g. is their angina worse recently, is their insulin-dependent diabetes well controlled?
- Current medications (as discussed later)
- Vital observations:
  - Pulse, BP, oxygen saturations, respiratory rate, blood glucose level if diabetic, and urine output in the trauma setting (urethral catheter)
- Investigations (refer to national guidelines and/or local guidelines for indications):
  - Urinalysis
  - Bloods, including group and save/cross-match
  - ECG +/– echocardiography
  - CXR
  - MRSA screen
- Full assessment of the affected limb for level of function, neurovascular status, concurrent infection and current analgesic requirements.

Medications (Chapter 8)

Some drugs may need to be discontinued or altered prior to surgery, whilst it is essential that others are continued throughout the perioperative period. Senior advice on this matter, from the surgeon, anaesthetist or specialist physicians, will often need to be sought as the risk/benefit balance is patient dependent. Protocol may differ depending on the urgency of surgery. Some examples to consider are:

- Aspirin and clopidogrel:
  - May need to be withheld prior to surgery because of bleeding risk (e.g. if a spinal anaesthetic is required).
- Warfarin:
  - Patients with heart valve replacements, recurrent DVT or PE may require conversion to intravenous heparin before the operation (discuss with haematology/cardiology)
  - Patients on warfarin for atrial fibrillation, low molecular weight heparin (LMWH) may suffice, with warfarin restarted postoperatively
  - Trauma patients may require reversal of warfarin with vitamin K or prothrombin complex concentrate
- Nephrotoxic drugs, e.g. ACE inhibitors and NSAIDs:
  - Patients susceptible to developing acute renal failure postoperatively may need some medications temporarily stopped and these will often be temporarily withheld postoperatively following major surgery

- Early catheterization to monitor urine output in certain groups of patients may be indicated
- Antihypertensives:
  - Patients will often have to remain on these medications for the operation, in particular beta blockers
- Steroids:
  - Patients on long-term oral steroids may require supplementation with increased doses of hydrocortisone perioperatively to avoid an Addisonian crisis
  - A local protocol regimen will often be available
- Consider an insulin sliding scale for diabetic patients (often mandatory when fasting in IDDM):
  - Depends on whether a short or long fast is expected.

It is important to consider prophylaxis for avoidable complications preoperatively (patient, operation and injury dependent):

- Antibiotics:
  - Refer to local guidelines for current indications
  - If metalwork is being placed one preoperative dose is usually given, with two postoperative doses (8 and 16 hours) dependent on the surgery
- DVT/PE:
  - Well hydrated, good pain relief and early mobilization
  - Mechanical prophylaxis, e.g. compression stockings (if there are no contraindications) and foot pumps
  - Chemical prophylaxis, e.g. subcutaneous LMWH, aspirin and warfarin.

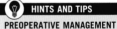

HINTS AND TIPS

PREOPERATIVE MANAGEMENT

Patients on long-term steroids may need increased doses perioperatively to avoid an Addisonian crisis. Effective VTE prophylaxis requires both mechanical and chemical methods. It is important to determine any personal or family history for VTE to help stratify the risk for the patient. Scoring systems are available to aid with this. Many hospitals perform as standard a VTE risk-assessment for all in-patients.

POSTOPERATIVE MANAGEMENT

Regular monitoring of vital observations (pulse, BP, urine output, respiratory rate, oxygen saturation, temperature) and blood tests are an essential part of immediate postoperative care. The Scottish Early Warning Scoring (SEWS) chart is an example of an effective way of identifying ill patients. Immediate assessment of the complications listed above will include:

- Bloods, e.g. for anaemia, renal and hepatic failure, infection
- ABGs, e.g. to determine hypoxia or degree of acidaemia/alkalemia
- ECG, e.g. for signs of myocardial ischaemia or dysrhythmia

- CXR, e.g. for signs of consolidation or fluid overload
- Septic screen, e.g. sputum, urine and blood culture to determine the organism causing pneumonia.

System Management

Cardiovascular and Renal Assessment

- Patients should be warm and well perfused.
- Monitor for causes and signs of shock, e.g. hypovolaemia due to operative site bleeding or from the GI tract (often secondary to NSAIDs), sepsis or cardiogenic shock.
- Monitor fluid and electrolyte balance regularly (urine output >0.5 mL/kg/h).
- Patients with preexisting established renal disease should be on a strict fluid balance:
  - Important to remember other losses, e.g. drains and vomiting.
- Susceptible patients are those with preexisting IHD, cardiovascular risk factors, the elderly and those with chronic kidney disease.
- Potential complications include atrial fibrillation, myocardial infarction, pulmonary oedema, acute renal failure, urinary tract infection and urinary retention.

Respiratory Assessment

- Monitor for symptoms and signs of respiratory distress, e.g. pyrexia, productive cough, abnormal CXR, increasing respiratory rate and/or oxygen requirements.
- Susceptible patients are those with preexisting pulmonary disease, e.g. chronic obstructive pulmonary disease (COPD) and a background or risk factors for VTE.
- Potential complications include pulmonary oedema, PE, pneumonia, acute respiratory distress syndrome (ARDS), fat embolism and atelectasis.

Systemic Assessment

- Monitor for sepsis, systemic inflammatory response syndrome and disseminated intravascular coagulation (DIC) in severe cases.
- Nutritional intake should be monitored as soon as possible postoperatively, with advice sought early if calorie requirements are not being met.
- In relation to nutrition, postoperative ileus may complicate oral intake due to abdominal pain, distension and vomiting.

Operative Field Assessment

- Neurovascular assessment of the limb(s) operated on
- Wound assessment including any drains
- Swelling
- Postoperative radiographs
- Early physiotherapy and occupational therapy input.

Analgesia Assessment

- Analgesic ladder (see Chapter 8)
- Some patients will require strong analgesia, e.g. morphine patient-controlled analgesia or epidural.

HINTS AND TIPS

POSTOPERATIVE MANAGEMENT

Observation charts and scoring systems are invaluable. Recognition of a deteriorating trend is as important as the actual numbers. Early specialist guidance and higher levels of care, e.g. critical care, may be required to deal with sick patients that may have potentially life-threatening complications. Nephrotoxic medications, in particular ACE inhibitors, should be temporarily stopped in the postoperative period to avoid precipitating hypotension and renal failure. In elderly patients particularly, always be vigilant for acute delirium or signs of opiate toxicity. Naloxone is an opioid antagonist that is used in the reversal of opiate toxicity.

FRACTURE COMPLICATIONS

Fracture Healing

The general aims of fracture management include pain relief, restoration of anatomy and optimization of function through early mobilization of the joint. There are numerous other significant complications (Table 4.5) that may occur with or without operative intervention.

The fracture healing process takes approximately 8–10 weeks (less in children):

1. Fracture haematoma
2. Inflammation (vascular invasion, inflammatory mediators and granulation tissue)

TABLE 4.5

COMPLICATIONS OF FRACTURES AND WHEN THEY COMMONLY OCCUR POSTINJURY

	Complications
Immediate	Neurovascular compromise
	Soft tissue injury
	Organ injury due to hypovolaemia (e.g. bleeding)
Early	Infection, e.g. at wound site, LRTI, ARDS
	Renal dysfunction, e.g. urinary retention or failure
	Cardiovascular, e.g. myocardial infarction, cardiac failure
	Emboli, e.g. DVT, PE, fat embolus
	DIC
	Fracture related, e.g. nerve damage due to poor cast position, failure of reduction, compartment syndrome
Delayed	Osteoarthritis (OA)
	Avascular necrosis
	CRPS
	Heterotopic Ossification (HO)
	Malunion, nonunion, deformity, stiffness and contracture

LRTI, lower respiratory tract infection.

3. Repair (subperiosteal osteoblast stimulation, endochondral and intramembranous ossification, bone matrix formation)
4. Remodelling (fusiform callus → woven bone → lamellar bone).

Fractures can heal by primary or secondary bone healing:

- Primary bone healing without callus formation: fracture is reduced anatomically and absolute stability is achieved with no motion at the fracture site. The bone remodels, via the cutting cones theory, which bridges the fracture site and lamellar bone is laid down.
- Secondary bone healing with callus formation: relative stability at the fracture site (a small degree of motion occurs).

Complications of Fracture Healing

Radiological union is often defined by the bridging of 3 of 4 cortices at the fracture site derived from combined AP and lateral radiographs. Complications of fracture healing are often related to fracture, patient and treatment factors (Table 4.6). Problems with healing are often categorized as:

- Delayed union: a fracture that takes longer than expected to unite due to organic insufficiency (e.g. poor vascular supply due to compartment syndrome, soft tissue injury or infection) or mechanical insufficiency (inadequate stability).
- Malunion: here the fracture has healed and the bone is united, but not in the correct anatomical position due to displacement (shortening, translation, rotation or angulation) and/or poor management of the fracture position:
  - Depending on the location and degree of mal-alignment, subsequent cosmetic deformity may be of no functional consequence.
- Nonunion: nonunited fracture results if the healing process has been unsuccessful with no clinical or radiological signs of fracture healing. Types of nonunion include:
  - Atrophic: no callus/bone formation, thinning of bone ends, often associated with a poor blood supply

---

TABLE 4.6

RISK FACTORS FOR DELAYED OR NONUNION, CATEGORIZED ACCORDING TO PATIENT, INJURY AND MANAGEMENT FACTORS

Patient Factors	Injury Factors	Management Factors
Age	Open fracture	Prolonged immobilization
Smoking	Extensive soft tissue trauma	Poor fracture reduction
Diabetes mellitus	Infection	Poor fracture fixation
Medications, e.g.	Neurovascular injury	
NSAIDs	Site of fracture (diaphysis/metaphysis)	
	Degree of bone loss	
	Polytrauma, e.g. head injury speeds callus	
	Pathological fracture	
	Fracture adjacent to a stiff joint	

Adapted from Datta PK, Bulstrode CJK, Wallace WFM. MRCS Part A: 500 SBAs and EMQs. JP Medical Ltd; 2013.

- Hypertrophic: abundant callus/bone formation with expansion of bone ends but no bridging at the fracture site, often associated with fracture motion and lack of stability at the fracture site
- Infected: fracture union inhibited by infection, which is a serious complication that can require multiple interventions and multistage treatment.

Fat Embolism

A rare complication that usually occurs following a long bone fracture, e.g. femoral shaft.

Pathogenesis

Two possible causes are:

1. Direct embolization of lipid globules (microemboli) from bone marrow adipocytes of the medullary canal at the fracture site to the end blood vessels in organs throughout the body.
2. Metabolic: altered response of lipid metabolism secondary to injury, which generates numerous small fat particles and activates the clotting cascade, ultimately resulting in endothelial vascular damage.

Presentation

Peak onset is 24–72 hours following injury. Signs depend on the end organ affected and include:

- Cardiorespiratory: shortness of breath, hypoxia, tachycardia and ARDS
- CNS: confusion, delirium, seizures and coma
- Renal: acute renal failure
- Ophthalmology: subconjunctival or retinal changes
- Systemic: petechial haemorrhagic rash (axilla/chest wall) and pyrexia.

Investigations

- Bloods (anaemia and thrombocytopenia)
- Urine and sputum analysis (lipids may be seen)
- ABG (low PO_2)
- CXR (pulmonary oedema and peripheral patchy consolidation).

Management

Treatment is with high positive end-expiratory pressure (PEEP) ventilation, steroids, intravenous fluids and organ support. The major complication is ARDS with a mortality rate of 10–15%. Risk of fat embolism is reduced by early stabilization of the fracture.

Acute Compartment Syndrome

Acute compartment syndrome occurs when the pressure within a confined fascial compartment increases beyond a critical level. This results in a decreased perfusion pressure to the compartment tissues, which without urgent diagnosis and treatment will lead to ischaemia and necrosis of the tissues.

Pathogenesis

Injured tissue expands due to oedema, haemorrhage and inflammation. As there is limited space within the enclosed fascial compartment, intracompartmental pressure rises, vascular (arterial and venous) flow is impaired, and the tissue (muscle and nerve) becomes ischaemic and necrotic. With muscle this eventually causes fibrosis and permanent contracture of the muscle (e.g. Volkmann ischaemic contracture in the forearm).

Risk Factors

- Younger adults
- Males
- Tibial diaphyseal fractures
- High energy forearm fractures
- Soft tissue injuries:
  - Crush injuries, crush syndrome (as discussed later), drug overdose and anticoagulation therapy.

Presentation

Commonly presents with swelling and intense severe pain, which is refractory to analgesia, out of proportion and worse on passive stretch. Paralysis, paraesthesia, pallor and an absent pulse are very late signs and are associated with either a vascular injury or the late stages of a missed compartment syndrome that is associated with a very poor outcome, e.g. amputation.

Investigations

Compartment monitors to monitor intracompartmental pressures:

- Recommended for at risk patients
- Diagnostic if ΔP (pressure difference = diastolic blood pressure – intracompartmental pressure) is ≤30 mmHg for more than 2 hours.

Management

Early open surgical decompression fasciotomy.

Crush Syndrome

Crush injury leading to ischaemia and necrosis of muscle. Is not a complication of fracture but is a complication of trauma. Muscle damage leads to the release of myoglobin into the circulation due to muscle breakdown (rhabdomyolysis). This can lead to renal and potentially multi-organ failure.

Presentation

- Myoglobinuria, which darkens the urine
- Beware of compartment syndrome (see above).

Investigations

- Blood tests:
  - Raised creatinine kinase (CK) level (with hypovolaemia this may lead to acute renal failure), hyperkalaemia
- ABG:
  - Metabolic acidosis

- Coagulation:
  - DIC when severe.

Management

- Intensive organ support, aggressive intravenous fluids with strict fluid balance
- Diuretics and urine alkalization
- Dialysis if severe enough
- Amputation in severe crush injury.

Avascular Necrosis

When a fracture affects the vascular supply to a bone and/or joint, bone ischaemia and eventually osteonecrosis (avascular necrosis) occur. It is found commonly when the vascular supply of the bone originates from the medullary cavity. Avascular necrosis can occur in the absence of trauma (e.g. Perthes disease, steroids, alcohol excess, sickle cell disease, Caisson disease).

Common susceptible injuries are:

- A proximal pole scaphoid fracture as the vascular supply to the bone enters distally
- An intracapsular femoral neck fracture when the retinacular vessels that supply the head of the femur are interrupted (Figure 4.4)

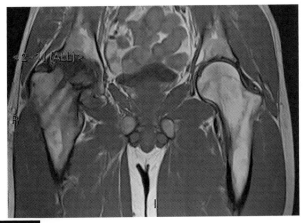

FIGURE 4.4

Coronal MRI demonstrating avascular necrosis of the right femoral head following previous cannulated screw fixation for a displaced intracapsular neck of femur fracture. *(Reproduced with permission and copyright © of the British Editorial Society of Bone and Joint Surgery. From Duckworth AD, Bennet SJ, Aderinto J, Keating JF. Fixation of intracapsular fractures of the femoral neck in young patients: risk factors for failure. J Bone Joint Surg [Br] 2011;93–B:811–816 (Figure 3).)*

TABLE 4.7

FICAT CLASSIFICATION OF FEMORAL HEAD AVASCULAR NECROSIS

Stage	Description
0	No diagnostic evidence on radiographs or MRI
1	Normal radiographs, but abnormal MRI
2	Sclerosis and cysts
3	Subchondral collapse (crescent sign), femoral head flattening
4	Joint space obliteration and advanced degenerative changes

- A neck of talus fracture as the vascular supply enters the bone via the talar neck.

Presentation

Patients present with:

- Stiff and painful joint with reduced mobility
- Onset can be rapid or chronic.

Investigation

- Radiographs: avascular fragment appears more dense than surrounding bone on a radiograph due to collapse, calcification and osteoporosis
- MRI
- Ficat classification (Table 4.7).

Management

- Analgesia and surgery (consider decompression and vascularized bone graft in early stages, joint replacement or fusion for established cases)
- AVN risk after fracture may be reduced by early reduction and definitive fixation.

 HINTS AND TIPS

FRACTURE COMPLICATIONS

The diagnosis of delayed union is dependent on characteristics of both the fracture and the patient. For example, an adult femoral fracture can take 12–16 weeks to unite, whereas a paediatric distal radius fracture will normally unite within 4 weeks. Clinical signs of compartment syndrome have a low sensitivity and specificity, whereas minimally invasive compartment pressure monitoring has been shown to have a high sensitivity and specificity for the diagnosis of acute compartment syndrome.

Chapter 5

Rheumatology and Bone Disease

CHAPTER OUTLINE

RHEUMATOID ARTHRITIS

 OVERVIEW

RA is the most common form of inflammatory arthritis. The typical presentation is with pain and stiffness affecting the small joints of the hands and feet. Early aggressive therapy aimed at suppressing inflammatory activity with DMARDs and biologicals has been shown to improve clinical outcome.

Rheumatoid arthritis (RA) affects all ethnic groups and the peak age at onset is between the ages of 60 and 75 years. The prevalence in Caucasians is about 1% and the female to male ratio is about 3:1.

Pathogenesis

The cause of RA is incompletely understood, but it is currently thought that genetically susceptible individuals develop the disease in response to environmental triggers, such as infections, that induce immune activation and cross-reactivity with endogenous antigens in the synovium and other tissues. There is a strong genetic association with the HLA variants DR4 and DR1, but also contributing are many other genetic variants of smaller effect size located close to cytokine genes and other genes involved in the immune response. Environmental triggers include smoking, which increases the risk of developing RA and its severity, and pregnancy, which has a protective effect. Histological analysis of affected joints showed inflammation of the synovium with an infiltrate of lymphocytes, polymorphs and macrophages with synovial hypertrophy. These cells release inflammatory cytokines including TNF, IL-1, IL-6, RANKL and other mediators that cause osteoclast activation and increase production of proteases that cause degradation of ligaments, tendons, bone and cartilage. Periarticular and generalized osteoporosis are common complications.

Presentation

The onset may be gradual or sudden. The characteristic features are:

- Pain, stiffness and swelling affecting the small joints of the hands, wrists, feet and other joints in a symmetrical fashion (Figure 5.1)
- Early-morning stiffness >1 hour
- Inactivity gelling (increased stiffness when patient has been inactive for a while)
- Synovial swelling and tenderness with an increased temperature over affected joints
- Joint deformity in longstanding disease (Figure 5.1)
- A clinical course of exacerbation and remissions.

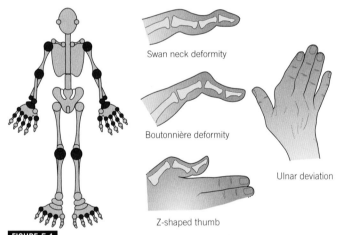

Swan neck deformity

Boutonnière deformity

Z-shaped thumb

Ulnar deviation

FIGURE 5.1

Deformities seen in RA hands. Ulnar and volar deviation of the finger joints due to synovial inflammation of the wrist and MCPJs. Wrist subluxation may lead to a prominent ulnar styloid. Tendon rupture, secondary to swelling of tendon sheaths and/or reported frictional trauma, can occur, e.g. extensors and flexor pollicis longus. Swan neck deformity is due to PIPJ hyperextension, with MCPJ and DIPJ flexion. FDS rupture or extensor digitorum shortening will lead to a similar presentation. Boutonnière deformity is due to a deficiency of the extensor tendon central slip leading to DIPJ hyperextension and PIPJ flexion.

TABLE 5.1	
DIAGNOSTIC CRITERIA FOR RA*	
Joints Affected	**Score**
1 large joint	0
2–10 large joints	1
1–3 small joints	2
4–10 small joints	5
Serology	
Negative RF and ACPA	0
Low positive RF or ACPA	2
High positive RF or ACPA	3
Duration of Symptoms	
<6 weeks	0
>6 weeks	1
Acute Phase Reactants	
Normal CRP and ESR	0
Abnormal CRP or ESR	1
Patients with a score ≥6 are considered to have definite RA	

*ARA / EULAR 2010 diagnostic criteria.

Diagnostic Criteria

Points are given for individual clinical features and if the score exceeds six the diagnosis of RA is confirmed (Table 5.1).

Extraarticular Features

Patients with RA often exhibit extra-articular features. These are most common in patients who are ACPA or RF positive. They include:

- Fever, fatigue and weight loss
- Rheumatoid nodules
- Scleritis and keratoconjunctivitis
- Dry eyes and dry mouth (Sjögren syndrome)
- Pericarditis and pleurisy
- Pulmonary fibrosis and lung nodules
- Anaemia
- Amyloidosis (rare)
- Vasculitis (rare)
- Felty syndrome (rare), comprising splenomegaly, leukopenia, lymphadenopathy, anaemia and thrombocytopenia.

Investigations

- Routine bloods: normochromic normocytic anaemia, thrombocytosis, raised ESR, raised CRP, mildly raised ALP
- Immunology: positive ACPA and/or RF positive (70–75%), ANA positive (50%) (see Chapter 3)

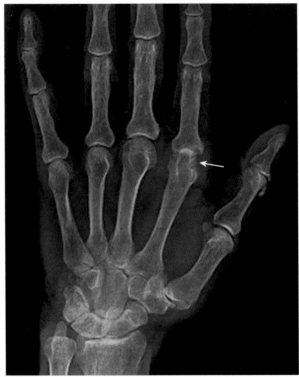

FIGURE 5.2

Radiograph of RA hand showing periarticular osteoporosis of MCPJs and an erosion of the first MCPJ (arrow).

- Synovial fluid: sterile, and cloudy with a raised WCC and low viscosity
- Imaging: periarticular osteoporosis and erosions on X-ray (Figure 5.2). Ultrasound and MRI are not routinely required but may be helpful in detecting subclinical synovitis and early erosions that are not evident on X-ray. If clinical risk factor analysis suggests a 10-year fracture risk of ≥10%, DEXA is indicated to check for osteoporosis.

Management

A multidisciplinary team approach is required involving pharmacological and nonpharmacological measures. Activity of RA is usually assessed using the DAS28 score. This involves examining 28 joints in the upper limbs and knees and counting the number that are swollen and tender (Figure 5.3); asking the patient to grade the activity of their arthritis on a scale of 0 (best possible) to 100 (worst possible); and measuring the ESR. This data is entered into a

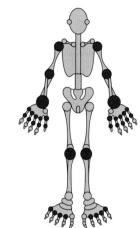

- Count swollen joints
- Count tender joints
- Ask patient about activity of arthritis (0-100)
- Measure ESR
- Enter data into calculator

Disease activity
- Remission   <2.6
- Low   2.6–3.2
- Moderate   3.2–5.1
- High   >5.1

FIGURE 5.3

Calculation of the DAS28 score.

calculator (http://www.das-score.nl). A smart phone app. is also available. Scores of <3.2 indicate low disease activity; scores between 3.2 and 5.1 indicate moderate disease activity; and scores >5.1 indicate high disease activity.

DRUG TREATMENT

On making the diagnosis of RA, DMARD therapy should be initiated early because this protects against joint damage and improves quality of life. A 'treat to target' approach is used aimed at lowering the DAS28 score. The core drug is methotrexate (MTX), which is often used in combination with a short course of corticosteroids at first diagnosis, but additional drugs may be added in a stepwise manner depending on disease severity and clinical response. A typical protocol for patients with early RA is as follows:

- MTX 10 mg/week, increasing gradually to 25 mg/week until synovitis is controlled (or side effects occur)
- Folic acid 5 mg daily the day after MTX (reduces haematologic toxicity and risk of some other side effects)
- Prednisolone 30 mg/day gradually reducing in dose over 12 weeks
- Low-dose maintenance oral steroids (5–10 mg daily) may be used longer term for patients who have an inadequate response to DMARDs and/or biological therapy
- Intraarticular steroids for problem joints and intramuscular steroids for disease flares
- Leflunomide (10–20 mg/day) can be used as an alternative to MTX
- Sulfasalazine and/or hydroxychloroquine can be added to MTX or leflunomide if the response is inadequate.

BIOLOGICAL THERAPIES

- Inhibitors of TNF (TNFi) are first line for inadequate response to DMARDs if DAS28 >5.1.
- Tocilizumab is first line in patients with DAS28 >5.1 who are MTX intolerant or in whom MTX is contraindicated.
- Alternative biologicals for TNFi failure include abatacept (inhibits T-cell activation), tocilizumab (anti-IL6) or rituximab (anti-B-cell therapy). Anakinra (IL-1 decoy receptor) is occasionally used.

PAIN RELIEF

Control of inflammation helps inflammatory pain but NSAIDs/analgesics may also be required in patients with mechanical damage (Chapter 8).

NONPHARMACOLOGICAL APPROACHES

- Education and joint protection strategies
- Splints, appliances and household aids
- Rest during disease flares
- Physiotherapy to encourage joint movement and maintain muscle power.

SURGERY

Has an important role in patients with mechanical damage to joints or tendons or when response to optimal medical management is inadequate. Procedures include:

- Joint replacement surgery:
  - Hip, knee, shoulder, elbow and MCPJs of hand
- Tendon repair or transfer
- Synovectomy
- Arthrodesis (e.g. wrist fusion), excision (e.g. ulna head excision) and osteotomy (seldom used).

Prognosis

Patients who are untreated and those who do not respond adequately have radiological signs of erosions and joint space narrowing within 2 years. Historical data show that life expectancy is decreased (~10 years for women, ~4 years for men), due to an increased risk of cardiovascular disease. There is some evidence that life expectancy has improved in RA over recent years, possibly due to better control of inflammation. Poor prognostic features are:

- Positive for ACPA and/or RF
- Extraarticular features
- Female gender.

 HINTS AND TIPS

RHEUMATOID ARTHRITIS

Rheumatoid patients are frequent exam cases. Early-morning stiffness is a classical symptom. Patients who are positive for ACPA have a worse prognosis. The use of aggressive therapy for RA means that the requirement for orthopaedic surgery has declined, but surgery still plays an important role in those who have progressive disease despite treatment.

SERONEGATIVE SPONDYLOARTHROPATHIES

 OVERVIEW

This is the term given to a group of inflammatory joint disorders that have overlapping clinical features. These disorders differ from RA in that:

- Tests for ACPA and RF are negative
- Joint involvement is usually asymmetrical
- Inflammation occurs at sites of tendon insertions (enthesopathy) and in fibrocartilaginous joints (sacroiliitis and spondylitis)
- New bone formation is a prominent feature
- There is a strong genetic association with HLA-B27
- Extraarticular features are distinct from RA

Ankylosing Spondylitis

Ankylosing spondylitis (AS) is a chronic inflammatory disorder characterized by inflammation and erosion of the SI joints and inflammation of the ligament insertions in the spine. This leads eventually to calcification of ligaments and bony fusion of the spine and SI joints. The diagnosis of AS can be made in a patient with low back pain and stiffness where there is radiographic evidence of sacroiliitis. The term 'axial spondyloarthropathy' has been introduced to describe the same condition but at an earlier stage, before radiographic evidence of erosions or ligament calcification has occurred. The onset of AS is usually during early adulthood (age 15–30) and the disease is more common in men (3:1). The population prevalence is about 0.15%.

Pathogenesis

The pathogenesis of AS is incompletely understood, but there is a strong genetic component and more than 90% of patients are positive for the HLA-B27. It is thought that HLA-B27-positive individuals develop the disease in response to an infectious trigger that causes immune activation and cross-reactivity with endogenous antigens. With progression of AS there is calcification of the affected ligaments and joints leading to the replacement of spinal ligaments and SI joints by bone.

Presentation

Low back pain and stiffness that is worse in the morning, and which improves with exercise. Diminished range of spinal movement in all directions leading to:

- Loss of lumbar lordosis
- Stooped posture with hyperextension of neck
- Flexion at hips and knees
- Diminished chest expansion
- Plantar fasciitis and Achilles tendonitis.

Diagnostic Criteria

Diagnostic criteria have been published for classical AS and axial spondyloarthropathy (Table 5.2) which can be considered to be an early form of AS.

TABLE 5.2

DIAGNOSTIC CRITERIA FOR AXIAL SPONDYLOARTHROPATHY*

The diagnosis of axial spondyloarthritis can be made in a patient with sacroiliitis on imaging and one other clinical feature in Table 5.2, or in a patient who is HLA-B27 positive with two other features.

Imaging

Sacroiliitis on MRI or X-ray

History

Back pain >3 months which has at least four of the following characteristics:
- improved by exercise
- not relieved by rest
- insidious onset
- night pain
- age at onset <40 years

Good response of back pain to NSAID

Family history of spondyloarthritis

History of inflammatory bowel disease

Examination

Arthritis

Enthesitis

Uveitis

Dactylitis

Psoriasis

Investigations

HLA-B27 positive

Elevated CRP

*Assessment of SpondyloArthritis international Society (ASAS) 2011 criteria.

Extraarticular Features
- Uveitis
- Aortic incompetence
- Restrictive ventilatory defects.

Investigations
- Routine bloods: normochromic normocytic anaemia, thrombocytosis, raised ESR and raised CRP. Normal results do not exclude diagnosis
- Immunology: autoantibodies negative
- Synovial fluid: sterile, and cloudy with a raised WCC and low viscosity
- Imaging: radiographs show erosions of SI joints; syndesmophytes; vertebral 'squaring' (loss of concavity of anterior vertebral bodies on lateral view due to erosions); calcification at entheses; and vertebral fractures. If clinical suspicion of AS is high and X-rays are negative MRI is indicated; typical features are erosions and bone marrow oedema around SI joints and inflammation at entheses.

Management
A multidisciplinary team approach is required involving pharmacological and nonpharmacological measures. Activity of AS is assessed by the Bath

ankylosing spondylitis disease activity index (BASDAI) score (www.basdai.com) in which patient-reported symptoms are recorded across seven domains. Scores of >4.0 indicate high disease activity.

DRUG TREATMENT

The first line treatment is NSAIDs supplemented by analgesics if necessary. Two different NSAIDs should be tried, each for at least 3 months, before progressing to biologic therapy:

- TNFi therapy for patients who respond inadequately (BASDAI >4.0)
- DMARDs (MTX or sulfasalazine) for peripheral joint arthritis (ineffective in spinal disease)
- Corticosteroids:
  - Oral steroids for uveitis
  - Intraarticular steroids for problem joints
  - Local steroid injections for plantar fasciitis and enthesitis.

NONPHARMACOLOGICAL TREATMENT

- Physiotherapy
- Education
- Back exercises.

SURGERY

- Joint replacement surgery (hip and knees)
- Spine osteotomy for severe deformity (technically challenging, high rate of complications and rarely performed).

PROGNOSIS

- Generally good
- Most patients (75%) remain in employment
- Lifespan normal.

HINTS AND TIPS

ANKYLOSING SPONDYLITIS

Low back pain with early-morning stiffness that improves during the day is the cardinal feature. Imaging with MRI is the most sensitive way of picking up early disease. Standard treatment is with NSAIDs, progressing to anti-TNF therapy in those who do not respond adequately.

Psoriatic Arthritis

Psoriatic arthritis (PsA) is an inflammatory arthritis that affects about 7% of patients with psoriasis. The arthritis usually occurs after the onset of psoriasis (70%) but can antedate the skin disease (25%), or present at the same time (5%). The disease predominantly involves synovial joints but some patients also have sacroiliitis and other features of AS. The overall population prevalence is about 0.5% and the peak age at onset is between 25 and 40. Males and females are affected equally.

Pathogenesis

Like other inflammatory joint diseases, PsA is thought to be caused by an infectious trigger in a genetically susceptible individual. There is a genetic association with variants in the HLA class I region, most notably HLA-C and with variants close to various cytokine genes and other genes involved in regulating immune function. Patients with spinal disease are usually HLA-B27 positive. There is an inflammatory infiltrate in affected joints as described for RA with increased production of TNF, IL-23, IL-12 and other inflammatory cytokines leading to bone, cartilage and soft tissue damage.

Presentation

A variety of presentations may occur:

- Asymmetrical inflammatory arthritis affecting PIPJ and DIPJ of the hands and feet. Large joints may also be affected (40%) (Figure 5.4)
- Symmetrical polyarthritis, similar to RA, but nodules and serological features of RA absent (25%)
- Dactylitis: predominantly targets PIPJ and DIPJ; and is strongly associated with nail dystrophy and pitting (15%)
- Psoriatic spondylitis: similar to AS with or without peripheral joint involvement in one or more of the patterns described above (20%).

Extraarticular Features

- Uveitis
- Psoriatic skin rash
- Nail pitting and nail dystrophy.

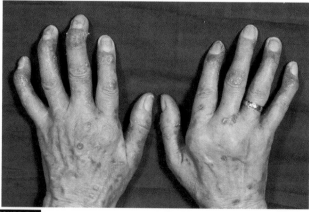

FIGURE 5.4

Asymmetrical arthritis involving the DIPJs and MCPJs of the hands with typical psoriatic skin rash.

Investigations

- Routine bloods: normochromic normocytic anaemia, thrombocytosis, raised ESR, raised CRP, and mildly raised ALP. Urate may be raised
- Immunology: autoantibodies negative
- Synovial fluid: sterile and cloudy with a raised WCC and low viscosity
- Imaging: bone erosions on X-ray. Ultrasound and MRI are not routinely required but may be helpful in detecting subclinical synovitis and early erosions that are not evident on X-ray.

Management

A multidisciplinary team approach is required involving pharmacological and nonpharmacological measures.

DRUG TREATMENT

More details on individual drugs are provided in Chapter 8. PsA has a better prognosis than RA so NSAIDs can be tried as a first-line treatment in mild disease.

- NSAIDs for mild disease
- DMARDs:
  - MTX first choice (helps skin and joints)
  - Leflunomide
  - Sulfasalazine
  - Combination DMARDs therapy may be used for resistant disease
  - Hydroxychloroquine contraindicated as can cause flare in skin disease
- Apremilast: inhibits phosphodiesterase D4 in leukocytes reducing inflammatory cytokine production. Effective in poor responders to traditional DMARDs. Recently licensed and role in therapy remains to be established
- Biological therapy: indicated in patients with ≥3 swollen and ≥3 tender joints despite DMARD therapy. Dactylitis (involvement of finger joints) only counts as one joint even though more than one digit may be involved
- TNFi therapy is first-line biological
- Ustekinumab (targets p40 subunit of IL-12 and IL-13) for TNFi-resistant disease.

PAIN RELIEF

Control of inflammation often improves pain but NSAIDs/analgesics may also be required for incomplete response and in those patients with mechanical damage to the joint.

NONPHARMACOLOGICAL APPROACHES

- Education and joint protection strategies
- Splints, appliances and household aids
- Rest during disease flares
- Physiotherapy to encourage joint movement and maintain muscle power.

SURGERY

Has an important role in patients with mechanical damage to joints or tendons or when response to optimal medical management is inadequate. Procedures include:

- Joint replacement surgery
- Tendon repair
- Synovectomy
- Arthrodesis and osteotomy (seldom used).

Prognosis

The prognosis of PsA is better than RA but up to 20% of patients develop joint damage. The incidence of cardiovascular disease in PsA is increased by about 50% compared with the general population. Treatment with DMARDs and biologicals can improve the quality of life significantly in patients with PsA in the short and medium term but the long-term effects have been less well researched.

 HINTS AND TIPS

PSORIATIC ARTHRITIS

The typical picture is of an asymmetrical arthritis affecting fewer joints than in RA. Many patients have mild disease and can be managed with NSAIDs, but DMARDs and biologicals may be required in those with active synovitis who do not respond adequately.

Reactive Arthritis

Reactive arthritis is an acute inflammatory arthritis that typically affects large joints in an asymmetrical pattern. It may occur as part of the Reiter triad of arthritis, urethritis and conjunctivitis. Males are predominantly affected (male:female ratio of 15:1) and the onset is typically between 15 and 40 years. The population prevalence is about 0.016%.

Pathogenesis

Reactive arthritis is thought to be caused by an infectious trigger in a genetically susceptible individual. The most important genetic risk factor is HLA-B27; about 95% are positive. The immune response to the precipitating infection is thought to result in cross-reactivity with endogenous antigens leading to acute inflammation in the joints and other affected tissues. Several weeks or months may elapse between the infection and onset of the arthritis. Recognized triggers include *Salmonella, Shigella, Campylobacter* and *Yersinia*, or sexually acquired infection with *Chlamydia*, but in many patients there is no obvious trigger.

Presentation

Reactive arthritis usually presents with an acute arthritis sometimes preceded by a diarrhoeal illness or urethritis. Clinical features include:

- Pain, stiffness and swelling of one or more large joints (often lower limbs)
- Heel pain, plantar fasciitis and Achilles tendonitis

- Nail dystrophy and keratoderma blennorrhagica (lesions similar to pustular psoriasis develop on soles and palms)
- Low back pain and stiffness.

Extraarticular Features

- Conjunctivitis (50%)
- Urethritis, circinate balanitis (ulcers and vesicles surrounding the glans penis) (15%)
- Mouth ulcers (10%)
- Uveitis (rare)
- Aortic incompetence, pericarditis, peripheral neuropathy and meningoencephalitis (very rare).

Investigations

- Routine bloods: raised ESR, CRP and thrombocytosis
- Synovial fluid: sterile, and cloudy with a raised WCC and low viscosity, and giant macrophage-like cells (Reiter cells) may be observed
- Imaging: radiographs may reveal sacroiliitis, syndesmophytes and ligament calcification at entheses in chronic disease
- Microbiology: *Chlamydia* on urethral or vaginal swabs, stool culture usually negative; serology may reveal evidence of previous gut infection.

Management

The aims are to treat synovitis of the affected joints and where appropriate to introduce DMARD therapy for recurrent or persistent disease:

- NSAIDs and analgesics are first-line treatment
- Intraarticular steroids or a short course of oral steroids for inadequate responders
- DMARD therapy:
  - MTX or sulfasalazine for persistent or relapsing disease
- Antibiotics:
  - Tetracycline for chlamydial urethritis.

Prognosis

Generally good but recurrence of arthritis in up to 60% of cases.

 HINTS AND TIPS

REACTIVE ARTHRITIS

The most important differential diagnosis is septic arthritis and it is important to aspirate the joint to exclude this possibility. Although reactive arthritis responds well to intraarticular steroids, these should not be given until infection has been excluded.

Enteropathic Arthritis

Approximately 15% of patients with IBD develop ankylosing spondylitis and/or a large joint asymmetrical peripheral inflammatory arthritis. If spine disease predominates, then management is as described for AS; if peripheral disease predominates, management is as described for PsA. Joint symptoms in IBD do not necessarily indicate enteropathic arthritis. A more common cause, especially in older people, is OA. Imaging for evidence of synovitis using MRI or ultrasound can help differentiate enteropathic arthritis from OA.

POLYMYALGIA RHEUMATICA

 OVERVIEW

Polymyalgia rheumatica (PMR) is characterized by pain and stiffness affecting the muscles of the shoulder and pelvic girdle. The prevalence increases with age and the mainstay of treatment is oral corticosteroids.

The onset of PMR is usually gradual with no obvious precipitating factor. It may present in isolation, or as a feature of giant cell arteritis (GCA) and many patients exhibit features of both conditions. Because of this, PMR and GCA can be considered to be different presentations of the same disorder. PMR is rare below the age of 50 but the prevalence rises from about 0.1% in those aged 55–60 years, to 3% above the age of 80. It is more common in females (1.7 : 1).

Pathogenesis

The cause is unknown, although some patients have a positive family history suggesting that there may be a genetic component. There can be evidence of tenosynovitis on imaging but no inflammatory infiltrate has been detected in affected muscles nor is there evidence of muscle vasculitis.

Presentation

- Proximal muscle pain and stiffness affecting pelvic and shoulder girdles
- Systemic upset (fatigue, malaise, anorexia, weight loss, low-grade fever)
- Headache and other symptoms suggestive of GCA may be present.

Investigations

- Routine bloods: normochromic normocytic anaemia, raised ESR, raised CRP and thrombocytosis, mildly raised ALP, and CK normal
- Immunology: autoantibodies negative
- Imaging: unhelpful.

Management

The aims of treatment are to improve symptoms and restore normal function. Oral corticosteroids are the treatment of choice. If symptoms do not improve substantially within 2–3 days then PMR is unlikely. A typical regimen is as follows:

- Prednisolone 15 mg daily for 3 weeks reducing to 12.5 mg for 3 weeks and 10 mg for 4–6 weeks.
- Reduce the prednisolone dose thereafter by 1 mg every month with the aim of eventually stopping treatment.
- If symptoms and raised ESR recur, increase the dose by about 5 mg for 2–4 weeks and then resume dose reduction.
- Most patients require 1–2 years of corticosteroid therapy; some require long-term treatment.

IMMUNOSUPPRESSIVES

Azathioprine (1–2 mg/kg/day) or MTX (10–25 mg/week) can be used as steroid-sparing agents in patients whose symptoms cannot be controlled on less than 10 mg prednisolone/day.

Prognosis

Generally good, but many patients require long-term corticosteroids and are at increased risk of adverse effects related to this treatment, especially osteoporosis.

 HINTS AND TIPS

POLYMYALGIA RHEUMATICA

Surgery in patients with PMR can be challenging as the result of osteoporosis secondary to long-term steroid use. The dose of steroid may need to be adjusted perioperatively to avoid an Addisonian crisis. Postoperative infection is a potential complication in those on long-term steroids.

GIANT CELL ARTERITIS

 OVERVIEW

Giant cell arteritis (GCA) is the most common primary vasculitis that affects the medium-sized vessels in the head and neck, including the ophthalmic and temporal arteries. Headache, jaw claudication and visual disturbance are classical features. A key aim of treatment is to prevent irreversible blindness.

In about 40% of cases it is accompanied by symptoms of PMR. It is rare under the age of 55 years, but like PMR becomes more common thereafter. The population prevalence of GCA above the age of 50 is about 0.025%, with a female : male ratio of 3 : 1.

Pathogenesis

The cause of GCA is unknown. Like PMR, some patients have a family history suggesting a genetic contribution. The disease is characterized by an inflammatory infiltrate of the affected vessels with destruction of the internal elastic lamina and granuloma formation with infiltration of macrophage-like polykaryons (giant cells). The lesions may be patchy in nature and affect only parts of the vessel wall (skip lesions).

Presentation

- Headache
- Temporal artery swelling and tenderness, with loss of pulsation
- Facial pain and jaw claudication
- Proximal muscle pain and stiffness affecting pelvic and shoulder girdle
- Visual disturbance, such as diplopia, amaurosis fugax
- Blindness due to involvement of ophthalmic, retinal and posterior ciliary arteries
- Systemic upset (fatigue, malaise, anorexia, weight loss, low-grade fever).

Investigations

- Routine bloods: normochromic normocytic anaemia, raised ESR (usually >50), raised CRP and thrombocytosis, and mildly raised ALP
- Immunology: autoantibodies negative
- Tissue biopsy: temporal artery biopsy can confirm the diagnosis but a negative result does not exclude GCA due to skip lesions. Treatment should not be delayed while awaiting biopsy
- Imaging: ultrasound and PET scanning being investigated but role in routine care not established.

Management

The aims of treatment are to prevent ocular complications such as blindness (which is irreversible) and to improve symptoms. High-dose glucocorticoids are the treatment of choice. If symptoms do not improve substantially within 2–3 days of starting corticosteroids then GCA is unlikely. A typical regimen is:

- Prednisolone >0.75 mg/kg (typically 40–80 mg daily) until symptoms respond and ESR falls (usually 4–6 weeks).
- Reduce by 10 mg every 2 weeks until a dose of 20 mg is reached.
- Reduce by 2.5 mg every 2 weeks until a dose of 10 mg is reached.
- Reduce by 1 mg every month depending on response and aiming to eventually withdraw treatment.
- Most patients require 1–2 years of corticosteroid therapy; some require longer-term treatment.

IMMUNOSUPPRESSIVES

Azathioprine (1–2 mg/kg/day) or MTX (10–25 mg/week) can be used as steroid-sparing agents in patients whose symptoms cannot be controlled on less than 10 mg prednisolone/day.

Prognosis

Good provided treatment is initiated quickly. Blindness when it occurs is irreversible. Corticosteroid-induced osteoporosis is a common complication unless prophylaxis is given (see Chapter 8).

 HINTS AND TIPS

GIANT CELL ARTERITIS

Treatment with steroids should not be delayed whilst awaiting a temporal artery biopsy. Although temporal artery biopsy is useful in confirming the diagnosis, false negative results are common due to skip lesions.

SYSTEMIC VASCULITIS

 OVERVIEW

These are a group of multisystem disorders characterized by inflammation and necrosis of blood vessel walls, and organ damage. The presentation is variable with many nonspecific symptoms and so a high index of suspicion is necessary to make the diagnosis. Immunosuppression with steroids and immunosuppressive drugs improve clinical outcome.

TABLE 5.3

THE CHARACTERISTIC FEATURES OF THE MAIN TYPES OF VASCULITIS

Type of Vasculitis	Main Sites Involved	ANCA Status	Comment
Takayasu arteritis	Aorta and major branches	Negative	Typically occurs age <50 years
Giant cell arteritis	Branches of carotid artery	Negative	Typically occurs age >50 years
Polyarteritis nodosa	Medium-sized arteries Aneurysms of visceral arteries	Negative	
Kawasaki disease	Large, medium and small arteries Coronary arteries may be involved	Negative	Usually effects children
Polyangiitis and granulomatosis	Small/medium-sized arteries in nasal passages, lungs and kidneys	Positive PR3	Also known as Wegener granulomatosis
Microscopic polyangiitis	Small arteries in lungs, skin and kidneys	Positive MPO	
Churg–Strauss syndrome	Small arteries in lungs	Positive MPO	Associated with asthma and eosinophilia
Henoch–Schönlein purpura	Small arteries in skin and kidney	Negative	Caused by IgA immune deposits in vessel walls
Cryoglobulinaemic vasculitis	Small arteries in skin and kidney	Negative	Caused by immune deposits (cryoglobulins) in vessel walls

This section covers the so-called primary forms of vasculitis but the condition can also occur in association with RA and SLE where it is thought to occur as the result of immune complex deposition in blood vessels. It is helpful to classify vasculitis by the size and type of vessel involved and the presence or absence of anti-neutrophil cytoplasmic antibodies (ANCA), which can be directed against myeloperoxidase (MPO) or proteinase 3 (PR3), which is summarized in Table 5.3. The individual types of vasculitis are discussed in more detail below.

Kawasaki Disease

This is a rare systemic vasculitis that predominantly affects children. It has long been considered to occur as the result of an infectious trigger but no specific organism has been isolated. With appropriate treatment the prognosis is good with complete resolution of symptoms and signs in most cases.

Presentation

- Febrile illness with systemic upset and lymphadenopathy
- Conjunctivitis; erythema of lips and mouth and tongue ('strawberry tongue')

- Erythema and swelling of hands and feet
- Skin rash and polyarthritis
- Cardiac involvement (pericarditis coronary artery aneurysms).

Investigations

- Routine bloods: normochromic normocytic anaemia, raised ESR, raised CRP and thrombocytosis, and mildly raised ALP
- Immunology: autoantibodies negative
- Imaging: angiography may reveal coronary artery aneurysms.

Management

The aims of treatment are to improve symptoms and prevent vascular complications. High-dose aspirin and intravenous immunoglobulins are the treatment of choice.

Takayasu Arteritis

This is a granulomatous arteritis that affects the aorta and its major branches. It is a rare disorder (prevalence 1–2/million population) that predominantly affects women aged 25–30 (female:male ratio of 50:1). It rarely presents above the age of 50 years.

Pathogenesis

Unknown.

Presentation

- Claudication in the upper limbs
- Diminished or absent pulses
- Carotid or subclavian bruits
- Visual disturbances
- Syncope, CVA and hypertension.

Investigations

- Routine bloods: normochromic normocytic anaemia, raised ESR, and raised CRP
- Immunology: autoantibodies negative
- Imaging: angiography can confirm the diagnosis by showing irregularity and narrowing of the affected vessels in the aortic arch.

Management

The aims of treatment are to improve symptoms related to vascular compromise by immunosuppressive therapy. High-dose oral steroids (prednisolone 1 mg/kg) along with azathioprine or MTX are used, with the response titrated against ESR and CRP, and clinical symptoms and angiographic findings. Hypertension should be treated if present.

Polyarteritis Nodosa

Polyarteritis nodosa (PAN) is a rare disorder with a prevalence of 30/million, which typically presents between 30 and 50 years of age. Men and women are affected with equal frequency and it is characterized by vessel wall necrosis and aneurysm formation, leading to thrombosis, infarction and bleeding.

Pathogenesis

In many cases the cause is unclear but there is a strong association with hepatitis B infection when the vasculitis is thought to occur as a result of deposition of immune complexes in the affected vessel wall.

Presentation

- Systemic upset (fever, weight loss, lethargy, myalgia, arthralgia)
- Peripheral neuropathy (mononeuritis multiplex)
- Abdominal pain and/or GI bleeding (mucosa ulceration, infarction)
- Acute renal failure, hypertension and haematuria
- Skin rash and skin ulceration (gangrene, nodules)
- Cardiac disease (MI, cardiac failure, pericarditis).

Investigations

- Routine bloods: normochromic normocytic anaemia, leucocytosis, thrombocytosis, raised ESR and CRP; ± raised urea and creatinine
- Urinalysis: haematuria
- Immunology: ANCA and autoantibodies negative; complement levels may be reduced
- Microbiology: serology for hepatitis B may be positive
- Imaging: angiography can be diagnostic in showing aneurysms of medium-sized vessels in the kidney, GI tract and other sites
- Tissue biopsy: necrotising vasculitis of medium-sized vessels. Helpful if angiography is inconclusive.

Management

The aims of treatment are to prevent organ damage and to reduce morbidity and mortality. High-dose steroids and immunosuppressives are used to induce remission, followed by low-dose steroids and immunosuppressives to maintain remission.

INDUCTION OF REMISSION

- Oral cyclophosphamide (2 mg/kg/day) or pulse intravenous cyclophosphamide for 3–6 months (as discussed later).
- The organosulfur compound mesna should be given during treatment with cyclophosphamide to protect the bladder from haemorrhagic cystitis.
- Oral prednisolone (1 mg/kg/day) for 1–2 months, gradually reducing to 10 mg daily or less by 6 months.
- One to three pulses of 1000 mg intravenous methylprednisolone at the start of treatment.
- Antiviral therapy for patients who are hepatitis B positive.

Pulses of intravenous cyclophosphamide can be used instead of oral cyclophosphamide. In this case a typical regimen of 15 mg/kg is given every 2 weeks for 3 cycles followed by further pulses of 15 mg/kg every 3 weeks for a further 3 to 6 cycles, depending on response.

MAINTENANCE OF REMISSION

- Azathioprine (1–2 mg/kg/day) after 6 months along with low-dose steroids
- MTX or mycophenolate can be used as alternatives to azathioprine.

Microscopic Polyangiitis

Microscopic polyangiitis (MPA) is a small vessel vasculitis that primarily targets the lungs (causing alveolar haemorrhage) and kidneys (causing rapidly progressive glomerular nephritis). The prevalence is about 150/million with a slight male preponderance.

Pathogenesis

The cause is unknown, but the pattern of occurrence is cyclical and possibly suggestive of an infectious aetiology or trigger.

Presentation

- Systemic upset (malaise, weight loss, fever)
- Renal impairment
- Haemoptysis and pleural effusions
- Skin rash and abdominal pain
- Neuropathy.

Investigations

- Routine bloods: normochromic normocytic anaemia, raised ESR, raised CRP, and raised urea and creatinine
- Urinalysis: proteinuria and haematuria
- Immunology: low complement; MPO-ANCA positive, ANA and anti-dsDNA negative
- Tissue biopsy: necrotising vasculitis of small vessels in renal, lung or skin biopsy.

Management

The aims of treatment are to prevent organ damage and to reduce morbidity and mortality. High-dose steroids and cyclophosphamide are used to induce remission, followed by low-dose steroids and azathioprine to maintain remission as described for PAN. Rituximab may be used as an alternative to cyclophosphamide during the acute phase, when it is given in a dose of 375 mg/m^2 body surface area once a week for 4 weeks along with high-dose corticosteroids. In contrast to cyclophosphamide-containing regimens, it is not necessary to introduce azathioprine or another immunosuppressive at 6 months in patients treated with rituximab because the immunosuppressive effect lasts for up to 18 months. Following this time it remains to be determined whether further rituximab or azathioprine should be introduced to maintain remission.

Granulomatosis with Polyangiitis

Granulomatosis with polyangiitis, also known as Wegener granulomatosis, is a small vessel vasculitis that involves the upper airways and nasal passages, lungs and kidneys. The prevalence is about 75/million; men and women are affected with equal frequency.

Pathogenesis

Unknown.

Presentation

- Epistaxis, nasal crusting, chronic sinusitis and mucosal ulceration
- Haemoptysis and dyspnoea

- Deafness due to serous otitis media
- Proptosis and diplopia
- Destruction of bone and cartilage in orbits nasal passages
- Renal impairment.

Investigations

- Routine bloods: normochromic normocytic anaemia, raised ESR, raised CRP, and raised urea and creatinine
- Urinalysis: proteinuria and haematuria
- Immunology: low complement; PR3-ANCA positive, ANA and anti-dsDNA negative
- Tissue biopsy: necrotising vasculitis with granuloma formation in small and medium-sized vessels in biopsy from kidney, lung or nasal passages.

Management

The aims of treatment are to prevent organ damage and to reduce morbidity and mortality. High-dose steroids and cyclophosphamide are used to induce remission, followed by low-dose steroids and azathioprine to maintain remission as described for MPA. Like MPA, rituximab can be used instead of cyclophosphamide to induce and maintain remission.

Eosinophilic Granulomatosis with Polyangiitis

Eosinophilic granulomatosis with polyangiitis, formerly known as Churg–Strauss syndrome, is a small vessel vasculitis that primarily targets the lungs but which can also affect the skin, gut, peripheral nerves and kidney. The prevalence is about 5/million; men and women are affected with equal frequency. About 40% of patients are ANCA positive.

Pathogenesis

Unknown.

Presentation

- Skin lesions with vasculitis rash or nodules
- Mononeuritis multiplex
- Allergic rhinitis and nasal polyps
- Dyspnoea and asthma-like symptoms that may be difficult to control
- Abdominal pain
- Glomerulonephritis.

Investigations

- Routine bloods: normochromic normocytic anaemia, leukocytosis, eosinophilia, thrombocytosis, raised ESR, CRP, and raised urea and creatinine
- Urinalysis: proteinuria and haematuria
- Immunology: low complement; MPO-ANCA or PR3-ANCA positive, ANA and anti-dsDNA negative
- Imaging: pulmonary infiltrates, pleural or pericardial effusions
- Tissue biopsy: necrotising vasculitis with eosinophil infiltrate and granuloma formation.

Management

The aims of treatment are to prevent organ damage and to reduce morbidity and mortality. High-dose steroids and cyclophosphamide are used to induce remission, followed by low-dose steroids and azathioprine to maintain remission as described for MPA.

Henoch–Schönlein Purpura

Henoch–Schönlein purpura is a small vessel vasculitis affecting the skin, gut and kidney that predominantly (75%) occurs in children. The prevalence is about 150/million with a slight male preponderance (1.5:1). It is usually self-limiting with a good prognosis.

Pathogenesis

The condition is thought to be caused by an infectious trigger which causes immune activation and overproduction of IgA which form immune complexes that become deposited in vessel walls, setting up an inflammatory reaction.

Presentation

The condition often follows an upper respiratory infection:

- Vasculitic skin rash over the buttocks and lower legs
- Abdominal pain and GI bleeding
- Arthralgia or arthritis
- Glomerulonephritis (can be delayed up to 4 weeks after other symptoms).

Investigations

- Routine bloods: raised ESR, raised CRP, and raised urea and creatinine
- Urinalysis: proteinuria and haematuria
- Immunology: negative
- Tissue biopsy: seldom required but skin or renal biopsy shows small vessel vasculitis with IgA deposition in the vessel wall.

Management

Henoch–Schönlein purpura is usually self-limiting and may not require treatment. In patients with persistent symptoms or signs, oral corticosteroids in doses of 1 mg/kg/day tapering rapidly over 2–4 weeks can be used.

Cryoglobulinaemic Vasculitis

This is a rare vasculitis that is caused by deposition of immune complexes in the vessel wall. The name stems from the fact that the antibody antigen complexes precipitate in low temperatures.

Pathogenesis

The vasculitis is thought to be due to immune complex deposition in blood vessels, which provokes a local inflammatory response. There is a strong association with infections particularly hepatitis C.

Presentation

- Systemic upset
- Vasculitis skin rash

- Neuropathy (mononeuropathy or polyneuropathy)
- Myalgia and arthralgia
- Raynaud syndrome.

Investigations

- Routine bloods: raised ESR and CRP
- Immunology: autoantibodies negative
- Cryoglobulin test: positive
- Microbiology: hepatitis C serology may be positive
- Tissue biopsy: vasculitis with immunoglobulin and C3 deposits in and around blood vessels.

Management

The aims of management are to improve symptoms and prevent organ damage. Management is empirical and lacks a good evidence base. High-dose corticosteroids, immunosuppressives and plasmapheresis have all been employed, with varying degrees of success.

Behçet Syndrome

Behçet syndrome is a vasculitis that can affect arteries and veins of all sizes. The highest prevalence is in Turkey where it affects about 0.4% of the population but it is also prevalent in other people of Mediterranean descent and Japanese descent. Males and females may both be affected.

Pathogenesis

The cause is incompletely understood but there is a strong genetic component and the condition is associated with HLA-B51.

Presentation

There is a wide range of clinical features:

- Oral and genital ulcers
- Uveitis and retinal vasculitis
- Erythema nodosum and acneiform lesions
- Arthralgia and arthritis
- Migratory thrombophlebitis and venous thrombosis
- Arterial aneurysms
- Aseptic meningitis and focal neurological lesions
- Pathergy reaction – development of a pustule at the site of skin trauma such as intradermal skin pricking with a needle.

Investigations

- Routine bloods: mild elevation in ESR and CRP, which correlates poorly with disease activity
- Immunology: autoantibodies negative
- Imaging: angiography may show evidence of venous thrombosis or arterial aneurysms. MRI may reveal evidence of cerebral vasculitis
- Lumbar puncture: increased WCC and protein with neurological involvement.

Management

Various treatments have been found to be effective in clinical trials as summarized below:

- Topical steroids for oral and genital ulceration
- Thalidomide (100–300 mg/day) for resistant oral and genital ulceration
- Colchicine (up to 1.2 g daily) for erythema nodosum and arthralgia
- High-dose steroids and immunosuppressives for neurological involvement as described for PAN.

ADULT-ONSET STILL DISEASE

This is a systemic inflammatory disorder that predominantly affects young adults between 20 and 40 years of age. It shares several clinical features in common with childhood Still disease.

Pathogenesis

There is some evidence for a genetic component and associations with the HLA locus have been reported but the studies have been small. An infectious trigger has been speculated but no specific organism has been identified.

Presentation

There are a wide range of clinical features:

- Intermittent fever
- Maculopapular skin rash
- Polyarthritis and polyarthralgia
- Myalgia
- Sore throat and lymphadenopathy
- Hepatosplenomegaly and abnormal LFTs
- Abdominal pain
- Pneumonia
- Liver failure (rare).

Investigations

- Routine bloods: elevated ESR and CRP, leukocytosis, thrombocytosis, and markedly elevated ferritin (10–20×upper limit of normal)
- Immunology: autoantibodies negative
- Imaging: lung infiltrates on CXR. Abdominal ultrasound may reveal hepatosplenomegaly.

Management

The aims of management are to improve symptoms:

- NSAIDs are first line for joint pains and fever
- Oral corticosteroids (40 mg prednisolone/day, reducing gradually)
- Azathioprine for incomplete responders (2 mg/kg/day)
- Various biological drugs including anakinra, canakinumab, tocilizumab and TNFi therapy have been used in patients who fail to respond to steroids and immunosuppressives.

HINTS AND TIPS

ADULT-ONSET STILL DISEASE

This often presents to infectious diseases units with a pyrexia of unknown origin, rash and arthralgia. High levels of ferritin are characteristic and an important diagnostic clue. Management is with steroids and immunosuppressives.

FAMILIAL FEVER SYNDROMES

These are a rare group of mainly inherited disorders that present with intermittent fevers lasting for a few hours up to several days in association with various other clinical features.

Pathogenesis

These are rare inherited disorders caused by mutations in various genes involved in immune regulation. The genes include *TNFRSF1A* (encoding the TNF type 1 receptor), *NALP3* and *MEFV* (both involved in processing and activation of IL-1β) and *MVK* (a gene involved in isoprenoid synthesis). In some cases no gene mutations have been identified.

Presentation

- Intermittent fever
- Skin rashes
- Arthralgia and arthritis
- Abdominal pain
- Serositis
- Conjunctivitis
- Amyloidosis.

Investigations

- Routine bloods: elevated ESR and CRP, raised IgD level (hyper-IgD syndrome), IgM paraprotein (Schnitzler syndrome)
- Immunology: autoantibodies negative
- Genetic testing: can confirm the diagnosis.

Management

NSAIDs can be useful for treatment of fever and arthralgia. Long-term colchicine is indicated in familial Mediterranean fever (caused by MEFV mutations). Anakinra and canakinumab have been successfully used in many of the syndromes.

SYSTEMIC LUPUS ERYTHEMATOSUS

 OVERVIEW

SLE is a multisystem autoimmune disease that can present in a variety of ways. It is characterized by the production of anti-DNA antibodies directed against double-stranded DNA and other components of the cell nucleus. Corticosteroids, hydroxychloroquine and immunosuppressive therapy are the mainstays of treatment.

Systemic lupus erythematosus (SLE) is a multisystem disease that can present with a wide variety of symptoms and signs. The peak age of onset is between 20 and 30 years of age and women are predominantly affected (10:1). The population prevalence is about 0.05% in the UK but the disease is about four times more common (0.2%) in people of Afro-Caribbean descent.

Pathogenesis

The cause of SLE is incompletely understood. There is a strong genetic component but environmental factors also play a role. A characteristic feature is the development of autoantibodies directed against DNA and other components of the cell nucleus. This has led to the hypothesis that there may be a defect in processing apoptotic cells in SLE, leading to inappropriate display of nuclear components on the cell surface and autoantibody formation. Environmental factors such as oxidative stress, infections and UV light exposure are important triggers and the disease can be drug induced (hydralazine, procainamide). Patients with inherited defects in components of the complement pathway (C1, C2, C4) run a greatly increased risk of developing SLE. There is also a polygenic component and associations with HLA-DR2, DR3 and several other candidate genes have been identified by genome wide association studies (GWAS).

Presentation

The clinical features of SLE are many, including:

- Polyarthritis or polyarthralgia
- Fatigue and malaise
- Photosensitive skin rash; alopecia with scarring
- Focal neurological signs, psychosis, seizures, depression, TIA and stroke
- Raynaud syndrome and livedo reticularis
- Mouth ulcers
- Haemolytic anaemia, leucopaenia, lymphopaenia and thrombocytopenia
- Glomerulonephritis and renal failure
- Pleurisy and pericarditis, pneumonitis and pulmonary fibrosis
- Myocarditis and sterile endocarditis
- Venous thromboembolism
- Recurrent miscarriages.

Diagnostic Criteria

Diagnostic criteria are summarized in Table 5.4. It is not uncommon to encounter patients who have some clinical features but who do not quite meet all the diagnostic criteria of SLE.

Investigations

- Routine bloods: anaemia, leukopenia, lymphopenia, thrombocytopenia, and raised ESR. Levels of CRP normal except during infections. U&E abnormal with renal disease
- Urinalysis: blood, protein or casts in renal disease
- Immunology: ANA positive (95–99%), anti-dsDNA (35%); tests for RF, ACPA, APA, anti-Ro, anti-La and Sm antibodies are positive in a proportion of cases; Coomb test positive in haemolytic anaemia. Low C3, C4 and CH50 levels during an acute flare or in patients with inherited deficiency

TABLE 5.4

DIAGNOSTIC CRITERIA FOR SLE

The diagnosis of SLE can be made in a patient with any 4 out of the 11 features whether these are present serially or simultaneously

Features	Characteristics
Malar rash	Fixed erythema, flat or raised, sparing the nasolabial folds
Discoid rash	Erythematous raised patches with adherent keratotic scarring and follicular plugging
Photosensitivity	Rash due to unusual reaction to sunlight
Oral ulcers	Oral or nasopharyngeal ulceration, which may be painless
Arthritis	Nonerosive, involving two or more peripheral joints
Serositis	Pleuritis (history of pleuritic pain or rub, or pleural effusion) or pericarditis (rub, ECG evidence or effusion)
Renal disorder	Persistent proteinuria >0.5 g/day or cellular casts (red cell, granular or tubular)
Neurological disorder	Seizures or psychosis In the absence of provoking drugs or metabolic derangement
Haematological disorder	Haemolytic anaemia or leucopenia[1] or lymphopenia[1] or thrombocytopenia[1] in the absence of offending drugs
Immunological disorder	Anti-DNA antibodies In abnormal titre or presence of antibody to Sm antigen or positive antiphospholipid antibodies
ANA disorder	Abnormal titre of ANA by immunofluorescence

[1]On two separate occasions.

- Imaging: no erosions on X-ray of affected joints; ultrasound or MRI may be normal or show synovitis; imaging of heart and lungs may show pulmonary fibrosis, valvular disease and vegetations (Libman–Sacks endocarditis), pleural or pericardial effusions, and evidence of pulmonary embolus (patients with APA); neuroimaging may show white matter lesions, vasculitis or cerebral ischaemia (patients with APA)
- Lumbar puncture: increased white cells, protein and immunoglobulins in cerebrospinal fluid (CSF) with cerebral lupus
- Tissue biopsy: glomerulonephritis in renal SLE (a wide variety of patterns may occur). Skin biopsy may show deposition of IgG and complement in lesion.

Management

The aims of management are to control symptoms in mild/moderate lupus and to prevent organ damage and reduce morbidity and mortality in severe lupus.

SKIN AND JOINT DISEASE
- Hydroxychloroquine 200–400 mg/day
- Analgesics/NSAIDs for arthralgia and arthritis
- Low-dose oral steroids +/– azathioprine or MTX for patients who respond incompletely

- Avoidance of UV light and use of sunblock
- Topical steroid cream for discoid lupus
- Belimumab for patients resistant to standard therapy.

HAEMOLYTIC ANAEMIA
Oral corticosteroids +/– immunosuppressives.

THROMBOPROPHYLAXIS IN APA-POSITIVE PATIENTS
Low-dose aspirin (75 mg/day).

THROMBOTIC EVENTS IN APA-POSITIVE PATIENTS
Warfarin (INR 2.0–3.0).

RENAL, CARDIAC OR CNS INVOLVEMENT
Patients with significant renal, cardiac or neurological involvement require high-dose steroids and cyclophosphamide to induce remission and low-dose steroids and immunosuppressives to maintain remission. The regimen is as described for PAN. Mycophenolate mofetil has been found to give equivalent results to cyclophosphamide for inducing remission in SLE with renal involvement. Randomized trials have shown no significant benefit of rituximab in SLE. Belimumab has been found to be effective in SLE that is resistant to standard therapy, including patients with renal, cardiac and haematological involvement but has not been studied in CNS lupus.

Prognosis
Patients with mild disease have a good prognosis with an overall 10-year survival of greater than 85%.

 HINTS AND TIPS

SYSTEMIC LUPUS ERYTHEMATOSUS

Patients with SLE have a substantially increased risk of cardiovascular disease thought to be due to inflammatory damage to the endothelium. The most common causes of death are infection, renal failure and cardiovascular disease.

SCLERODERMA

 OVERVIEW

Scleroderma (or systemic sclerosis) is a connective tissue disorder affecting the skin, internal organs and vascular system that is characterized by progressive fibrosis and multiorgan failure. Cardiorespiratory involvement is common and is the leading cause of death in these patients.

The onset of scleroderma is usually between the ages of 20 and 50 years and women are predominantly affected (4:1). The population prevalence is about 0.02%. Two subgroups are recognized: diffuse cutaneous systemic sclerosis (DCSS) – accounting for about 30% of cases – in which life threatening lung, gut and renal involvement may occur, and limited cutaneous systemic sclerosis (LCSS) – accounting for about 70% of cases – in which major organ damage is less common and the prognosis is a little better. A further subgroup of patients with limited cutaneous systemic sclerosis is recognized in which Calcinosis, Raynaud syndrome, oEsophageal involvement, Sclerodactyly and Telangiectasia occur (i.e. the CREST syndrome).

Pathogenesis

The cause is unknown although the disease clearly has an immunological basis. Autoantibodies to DNA and other extractable nuclear antigens are common. A hallmark of the disease is fibrosis of the skin and other tissues with deposition of collagen and narrowing of arterioles and small arteries associated with intimal proliferation and an inflammatory infiltrate.

Presentation

- Severe Raynaud syndrome often with digital ulceration
- Skin fibrosis (sclerodactyly, microstomia)
- Telangiectasia
- Calcinosis
- Oesophageal dysmotility
- Muscle pain and weakness
- Pulmonary hypertension and pulmonary fibrosis
- Hypertension and renal failure
- Polyarthralgia and contractures
- Malabsorption.

Investigations

- Routine bloods: levels of ESR and CRP usually normal. CK may be increased in patients with myositis. U&E may be abnormal with renal disease
- Urinalysis: blood or protein with renal involvement
- Immunology: ANA positive (90%), anti-Scl-70 (30%), anticentromere antibody (50% overall, up to 90% in CREST)
- Imaging: ultrasound or MRI may be normal or show synovitis; imaging of lungs may show pulmonary fibrosis and echocardiogram pulmonary hypertension
- Pulmonary function tests: restrictive defect
- Cardiac catheterization: indicated in patients with evidence of pulmonary hypertension.

Management

The aims of management are to control symptoms and manage complications as they occur:

- Antihypertensive medication to control raised blood pressure
- Proton pump inhibitors and antireflux agents for oesophageal symptoms
- Vasodilators and heated gloves for Raynaud syndrome
- Antibiotics for infected digital ulcers and blind loop syndrome
- High-dose steroids and immunosuppressives for pulmonary fibrosis
- Prostacylin or bosentan for pulmonary hypertension (refer to specialist unit).

Prognosis

The prognosis in diffuse cutaneous systemic sclerosis is poor with a 10-year survival of 70%. Cardiovascular disease, renal failure and pulmonary hypertension are the commonest causes of death. Patients with limited cutaneous systemic sclerosis have a better prognosis with a 10-year survival of 82%.

POLYMYOSITIS AND DERMATOMYOSITIS

These are rare diseases characterized by an inflammatory infiltrate of the skeletal muscle that presents with muscle weakness. The population prevalence of both conditions combined is about 0.02% and women are more commonly affected (2:1).

Pathogenesis

There is evidence of a genetic component and associations with the HLA-locus have been reported. Inflammatory myositis may occur in isolation or as a feature of other autoimmune diseases like scleroderma, SLE and Sjögren syndrome or in association with underlying malignancy (20% of cases).

Presentation

Polymyositis presents with proximal muscle weakness and systemic features such as fever, weight loss and fatigue. Muscle pain may also occur. Involvement of the respiratory and pharyngeal muscles may lead to aspiration pneumonia and ventilatory failure. Pulmonary fibrosis occurs in up to 30% of cases. In dermatomyositis, the presentation is similar but with additional features of a maculopapular rash over the extensor surfaces of the PIPJs and other joints (Gottron papules) and a violet discolouration of the eyelids and periorbital oedema (heliotrope rash).

Investigations

- Routine bloods: levels of ESR and CRP raised; CK usually increased but normal levels do not exclude diagnosis
- Immunology: anti-Jo-1 positive (20%). Other autoantibodies are positive in patients with underlying SLE, scleroderma and Sjögren syndrome
- Electromyography: short-duration, polyphasic motor unit potentials with spontaneous fibrillation potentials
- Muscle biopsy: inflammatory infiltrate with muscle fibre necrosis and evidence of regeneration. Pulmonary function tests: restrictive defect in some cases.

Management

The aims of management are to improve muscle function and to detect and treat any underlying malignancy. A typical regimen is as follows:

- High-dose steroids (prednisolone 1 mg/kg/day) for 4–6 weeks (typically 60–80 mg)
- Gradually reduce prednisolone dose to between 7.5 and 10 mg daily over 4–6 months based on clinical response and CK levels

- Continue low-dose steroids and immunosuppressives (azathioprine, mycophenolate mofetil (MMF) or MTX) long term to maintain remission
- Intravenous immunoglobulin in patients with resistant disease
- Treat underlying malignancy if present.

SJÖGREN SYNDROME

Sjögren syndrome is an autoimmune disorder characterized by inflammation of the salivary and lachrymal glands. The population prevalence in the UK has been estimated as 0.4%. The typical age at onset is between 40 and 50 years and females are more commonly affected (9:1).

Pathogenesis

Sjögren syndrome may occur in isolation or may be a feature of other autoimmune diseases such as RA, SLE, autoimmune thyroid disease or primary biliary cirrhosis. Patients with Sjögren syndrome run a substantially increased risk of developing lymphoma.

Presentation

The presenting symptoms are related to reduced production of tears and saliva, but a diverse range of other features may occur including:

- Dry mouth
- Dry or 'gritty' eyes
- Conjunctivitis and blepharitis.

Other features include:

- Fatigue
- Raynaud syndrome
- Lymphadenopathy
- Renal tubular acidosis
- Peripheral neuropathy
- Features of associated disease.

Investigations

- Routine bloods: raised ESR, CRP and hypergammaglobulinaemia
- Immunology: positive ANA and RF (90%); anti-Ro (60%) and anti-La (30%)
- Schirmer test: wetting less than 5 mm in 5 minutes
- Biopsy: lymphocytic infiltrate on biopsy of lacrimal gland, lip or salivary gland.

Management

The aims of management are to improve symptoms. Immunosuppressives have not been shown to be of value:

- Hypromellose eye drops
- Oral hygiene and maintain good hydration
- Take liquids frequently
- Treat oral infections if they occur.

FIBROMYALGIA

 OVERVIEW

Fibromyalgia is a condition of unknown cause characterized by chronic widespread pain with multiple tender spots on palpation, fatigue and sleep disturbance. There is some evidence that it may be due to abnormal processing of pain signals in the CNS.

In patients with fibromyalgia, there is frequently a history of stressful life events in the recent past or during childhood. It is associated with low income, being divorced or separated and having a low educational status. Accompanying features include: depression, facial pain, IBS and sleep problems. The peak incidence is between 30 and 60 years, and it is more common in females (6:1). The population prevalence has been estimated to be 2–4%.

Pathogenesis

The pathogenesis is unknown but neuropsychiatric factors with abnormal central processing of pain signals are thought to be involved. There is evidence for a genetic component.

Presentation

- Widespread aches and pains
- Hyperalgesia with moderate digital pressure at multiple sites (Figure 5.5)
- Chronic fatigue
- Anxiety, poor concentration and depression
- Forgetfulness and tension headaches
- IBS
- Paraesthesia
- Increased frequency of adverse reactions to medication.

Investigations

- Routine bloods: normal
- Immunology: negative
- Imaging: normal.

Management

The aims of management are to improve pain with medication and promote self-help and coping strategies. A multidisciplinary team approach involving the occupational therapist, physiotherapist and clinical psychologist are of value:

- Amitriptyline
- Duloxetine
- Gabapentin
- Fluoxitene (can be combined with amitriptyline)
- Paracetamol or compound analgesics
- Disease education
- Acupuncture
- Occupational therapy and physiotherapy
- Cognitive behaviour therapy and mindfulness.

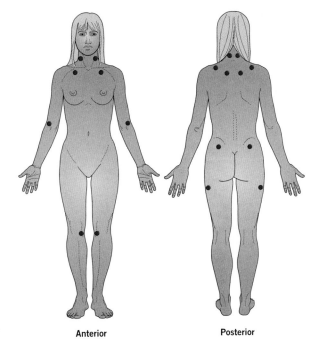

Anterior   **Posterior**

FIGURE 5.5

Regional tenderness in fibromyalgia.

Prognosis

In about 25% of cases, treatment results in an improvement of pain and about 50% of patients can continue to work.

COMPLEX REGIONAL PAIN SYNDROME

Two subtypes are recognized. Complex regional pain syndrome type 1 (CRPS1) which is discussed here is characterized by bone pain, localized osteoporosis and swelling of the affected limb with skin changes. It is thought to be due to a disturbance in neurovascular function, and often follows an episode of trauma. Complex regional pain syndrome type 2 describes the syndrome of neuropathic pain that follows a specific nerve injury.

Pathogenesis

The cause is unknown.

Presentation

- Pain persisting for weeks or months following injury
- Warmth, erythema and swelling of the affected area

- Local pain and tenderness
- Autonomic disturbance with skin atrophy and pallor of affected area.

Investigations

- Routine bloods: normal
- Imaging: patchy osteoporosis on X-ray. Local increase in tracer uptake on isotope bone scan; bone marrow oedema on MRI
- Bone biopsy: osteopaenia with no specific diagnostic features.

Management

The aims of management are to improve symptoms and restore normal function. Various drugs have been tried but the evidence base for their use is limited:

- Education
- Physiotherapy
- Analgesia:
  - NSAIDs
  - Antineuropathic agents
- Bisphosphonates.

Prognosis

Some patients improve spontaneously with time but many are left with permanent disability.

HINTS AND TIPS

COMPLEX REGIONAL PAIN SYNDROME

Complex regional pain syndrome type 1 may occur following fracture, as well as being associated with immobilization, and can delay recovery. Early and regular physiotherapy in combination with education are essential.

CRYSTAL-INDUCED ARTHRITIS

OVERVIEW

These are acute forms of arthritis caused by deposition of uric acid (gout) or calcium pyrophosphate (pseudogout) into the joints. Gout tends to affect younger people with a male predominance, whereas pseudogout more commonly affects older females. Synovial fluid microscopy can be helpful in making the diagnosis.

Gout

Gout is the most common form of inflammatory arthritis. There is a strong association with hyperuricaemia and metabolic syndrome. It most commonly presents in adults between the ages of 20 and 40 years and is more common in men (5:1). The population prevalence is about 2%.

Pathogenesis

Acute gout is caused by deposition of uric acid crystals in the joint, which sets up an inflammatory reaction. The underlying cause is raised levels of uric acid in the blood that can either be due to overproduction of endogenous uric acid or decreased urinary excretion. Genetic factors strongly influence rates of uric acid production and urinary excretion. A family history is not infrequent and some rare inherited conditions exist in which overproduction of uric acid occurs. Increased production of uric acid also occurs in myeloproliferative and lymphoproliferative disease and in psoriasis. Other important causes of hyperuricaemia include renal impairment, dehydration, excessive alcohol and thiazide diuretics.

Presentation

The presentation may be with an acute inflammatory arthritis or with a chronic arthritis interspersed with acute flares.

ACUTE GOUT

- Sudden onset of pain swelling, tenderness and redness typically affecting a single joint
- Most commonly targets the first MTPJ in the foot
- Other joints may be involved (lower limbs > upper limbs)
- Bursitis or tendonitis.

CHRONIC GOUT

- Soft tissue uric acid deposits (tophi)
- Chronic joint pain and swelling with intermittent flares
- Skin ulceration with extrusion of uric acid crystals
- Renal impairment.

Investigations

- Routine bloods: raised ESR and CRP, leukocytosis. Abnormal LFT due to coexisting metabolic syndrome or alcohol excess. Urate often raised but can be normal during acute attack
- Immunology: autoantibodies negative
- Synovial fluid: sterile, and cloudy with a raised WCC and low viscosity. Urate acid crystals often visualized
- Imaging: radiographs are usually normal in acute gout. In chronic gout, punched out erosions with periarticular osteosclerosis and joint destruction may be observed.

Management

The aims of management are to improve symptoms by treatment of synovitis during the acute attack and to institute urate-lowering therapy to prevent recurrences.

ACUTE ATTACK

- Colchicine 500 µg 2–3 times daily or NSAIDs
- Rest affected joints
- Intraarticular or systemic steroids in resistant cases.

LONG-TERM MANAGEMENT

- Allopurinol 50–100 mg daily and gradually increasing to 900 mg daily, titrated to reduce serum urate <360 µmol/L
- Febuxostat 80–120 mg in poor responders or allopurinol intolerance
- Reduce alcohol intake

- Avoid dehydration
- Avoid purine-rich foods (game, red meat, seafood).

Pseudogout

Pseudogout is an acute inflammatory arthritis associated with deposition of calcium pyrophosphate crystals in the joints. It is often associated with radiological chondrocalcinosis in which calcium pyrophosphate crystals become deposited in menisci and articular cartilage. There is also a strong association with OA. It most commonly presents in adults between the ages of 60 and 80 years and women are more commonly affected than men. The population prevalence of pseudogout has been estimated as about 0.5%.

Pathogenesis

Pseudogout is caused by precipitation of calcium pyrophosphate crystals in the joint, which sets up an inflammatory reaction. Deposition of calcium pyrophosphate crystals in articular cartilage is common and has been estimated to affect 7–10% of people aged 60 years. However, most patients are asymptomatic and only a few go on to develop pseudogout. Genetic factors play a role in determining susceptibility to pseudogout and in some cases the disease is familial and inherited in an autosomal dominant manner due to mutations in the *ANKH* gene. Chondrocalcinosis may also occur in association with other diseases including hyperparathyroidism, hypothyroidism, haemochromatosis, diabetes mellitus, Wilson disease and acromegaly. Recognized precipitating factors for an attack include surgery, trauma, dehydration, starvation and infection.

Investigations

- Routine bloods: raised ESR and CRP, leukocytosis. Urate normal
- Immunology: autoantibodies negative
- Synovial fluid: sterile, and cloudy with a raised WCC and low viscosity. Rhomboid shaped calcium pyrophosphate crystals may be visualized under polarized light but absence does not exclude the diagnosis
- Imaging: radiographs may show chondrocalcinosis and signs of OA (Figure 5.6).

Management

The aims of management are to improve symptoms by treatment of synovitis during the acute attack.

ACUTE ATTACK

- Colchicine 500 µg 2–3 times daily or NSAIDs
- Intraarticular or systemic steroids if patient fails to respond (providing sepsis excluded)
- Rest affected joints.

 HINTS AND TIPS

CRYSTAL-INDUCED ARTHRITIS

Serum urate falls during inflammation so a normal uric acid level does not exclude the diagnosis of acute gout. Both gout and pseudogout can mimic a septic joint and it is important to aspirate the joint so the correct diagnosis can be made.

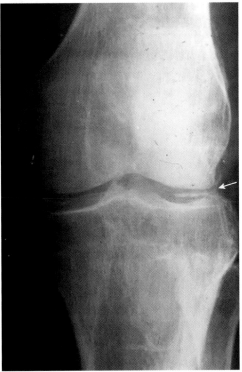

FIGURE 5.6

Chondrocalcinosis of the knee. This AP radiograph of the knee demonstrates calcification of the knee cartilage menisci due to crystal deposition in the lateral meniscus (arrow).

OSTEOARTHRITIS

 OVERVIEW

Osteoarthritis (OA) is the most common joint disease characterized by loss of articular cartilage in synovial joints and sclerosis of the subchondral bone. Radiographs are often diagnostic and treatment involves analgesia, exercise and lifestyle modifications. Joint replacement surgery is indicated when medical treatment no longer provides adequate symptom control and affects quality of life.

Osteoarthritis (OA) is characterized by cartilage damage and joint space narrowing with subchondral osteosclerosis and cyst formation. The knees, hips, hands and spine are the most commonly affected joints. Symptomatic OA is rare under the age of 50 but increases in frequency with age. It has been estimated that about 18% of people aged 55 in the UK have symptomatic knee OA, up to 4.4% have symptomatic hip OA and up to 2.5% have symptomatic hand OA. Radiological evidence of OA is even more common – about 80% of people over the age of 65 have evidence of the disease although most are asymptomatic. While OA runs a benign course in many individuals it is a major cause of morbidity and disability in older people.

Pathogenesis

Both genetic and environmental factors are involved in the pathogenesis of OA. A positive family history is common and twin and family studies have shown that heritability is substantial with a polygenic mode of inheritance. Biomechanical factors are important since OA is more common in occupational groups exposed to repetitive mechanical loading or joint injury. There is an association with increased bone density, and one theory of causation is that increased density of subchondral bone predisposes to OA by adversely affecting the shock absorbing properties of cartilage. There is a low-grade inflammatory component in some patients. Recognized risk factors for OA include:

- Family history
- Obesity
- Occupational damage to joints:
  - Professional sportsmen and women
  - Farmers
  - Miners
- Injuries:
  - Fracture affecting articular surface
  - Ligament rupture
  - Meniscal tear
- Coexisting disease:
  - Paget disease of bone
  - Septic arthritis
  - Congenital dislocation of the hip
  - Perthes disease.

Presentation

The typical presentation of OA is with joint pain that is worse on weight-bearing and relieved by rest (Table 5.5). There may be mild morning stiffness and inactivity gelling. Exacerbations and remissions occur. Characteristic features include:

- Anterior knee pain on descending stairs (patellofemoral OA)
- Pain at the base of the thumb (OA of first CMCJ)
- Hip or buttock pain on walking with limp (antalgic gait)
- Low-back pain or neck pain on movement (spine OA)
- Enlargement and bony swelling of affected joints due to osteophyte formation (Bouchard and Heberden nodes in the hands; Figure 5.7)
- Joint deformity:
  - Varus/valgus deformity of the knees
  - Fixed flexion deformity

TABLE 5.5

SPECTRUM OF PRESENTATIONS SEEN IN OSTEOARTHRITIS

Subtype	Features
Nodal OA	Nodal or primary generalized OA is less common, but has a strong genetic component that often affects women. It targets the PIPJs and DIPJs of the hands and first CMCJ at the base of the thumb. Patients may experience intermittent flares in symptoms due to local inflammation. Nodal OA of the hands is often associated with knee and hip OA, along with the first MTPJ (hallux rigidus)
Hip OA	Common in Caucasian populations, this category of presentation is often classified on the radiological appearance: superior-pole hip OA (common in men, unilateral, weight-bearing surfaces primarily affected) and medial cartilage loss (common in women, bilateral, coexists with nodal/hand OA)
Knee OA	More common in women and increases with age Strongly associated with obesity Other predisposing factors are previous knee trauma, e.g. such as meniscal, ACL and PCL tears Often a bilateral condition, with OA of the medial compartment of the knee leading to a bow-leg presentation, due to a bilateral varus deformity. Strong association with OA of the hand

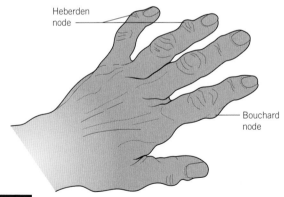

Heberden node

Bouchard node

FIGURE 5.7

Nodal OA with characteristic bony swellings. DIPJ involvement is known as Heberden nodes and PIPJ involvement as Bouchard nodes. Nodal OA has a propensity for the DIPJs over the PIPJs, commonly only affecting one joint at a time over a period of years. The presentation in the inflammatory phase is with pain, swelling and reduction of function in the affected hand. CMCJ and MCPJ involvement, particularly of the thumb, may coexist.

- Leg length discrepancy
    - Deformity of digits in hand OA
- Crepitus, decreased range of movement and muscle wasting
- Mild synovitis and effusion.

Investigations

- Routine bloods: normal
- Immunology: autoantibodies negative
- Synovial fluid: sterile, clear fluid with high viscosity; WCC may be slightly raised.
- Imaging: knee and hip X-rays should be taken whilst weight-bearing. Skyline and lateral views for patellofemoral OA. Typical features include loss of joint space, osteophytes, subchondral sclerosis and cysts (Figure 5.8).

Management

The aims of management are to improve symptoms. Pharmacological and nonpharmacological approaches are equally important:

DRUG TREATMENT

- Paracetamol
- Local NSAIDs

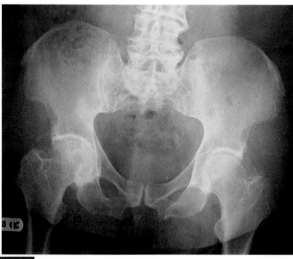

FIGURE 5.8

OA of the right hip. Changes include joint space narrowing due to loss of cartilage, subarticular sclerosis, subchondral cysts and osteophyte formation causing 'lipping' at joint margins. Pathological features of OA are subchondral cysts, bursitis, periarticular osteophytes, subchondral sclerosis, fibrillation and loss of cartilage, and synovial hyperplasia.

- Systemic NSAIDs
- Compound analgesics
- Intraarticular steroids.

NUTRACEUTICALS
Glucosamine/chondroitin (evidence for benefit is marginal).

NONPHARMACOLOGICAL APPROACHES
- Weight loss
- Quadriceps exercises in knee OA
- Disease education.

SURGERY
Indicated when medical management fails to control symptoms and quality of life is impaired:

- Total hip and knee replacement (see Chapter 6) is most successful
- Osteotomy (performed less commonly)
- Arthrodesis (occasionally performed).

Prognosis
Many patients can be successfully managed medically. Joint replacement surgery commonly gives good results but between 5% and 20% have a disappointing outcome in terms of pain response.

HINTS AND TIPS

OSTEOARTHRITIS

Can usually be differentiated from RA on clinical grounds and by the absence of erosions on X-ray, but sometimes both conditions can coexist. In this case the presence of synovitis and an acute phase response favours RA as a cause of joint pain and stiffness as opposed to OA. Radiographic changes do not always correlate with symptom severity. Avascular necrosis can occur in the late stages of OA. Weight loss and exercise are beneficial, whether or not joint replacement surgery is planned.

OSTEOPOROSIS

OVERVIEW

Osteoporosis is a common disease that increases in incidence with age. It affects women more often than men and is characterized by a low BMD, increased bone fragility and an increased risk of fracture. DEXA scanning plays a key role in the diagnosis and selecting patients for treatment. Bisphosphonates are the treatments of first choice.

Osteoporosis is defined to exist when BMD values are reduced by more than 2.5 standard deviations (T-score units) below the value observed in young healthy adults (see Chapter 3). The prevalence of osteoporosis increases with age and fractures related to osteoporosis are estimated to affect 30% of women and 12% of men at some time in their life. The current cost of treating osteoporotic fractures in the UK is estimated at about £1.2 billion and most of this is accounted for by hip fractures, which cause substantial morbidity and are associated with significant mortality.

Pathogenesis

The main cause of osteoporosis is increased bone loss associated with age and (in women) postmenopausal oestrogen deficiency. Both factors cause uncoupling of bone resorption from bone formation such that the amount of bone removed by osteoclasts (bone-resorbing cells) during remodelling of bone is greater than the amount replaced by osteoblasts (bone-forming cells). Ageing itself also plays a key role in the pathogenesis of osteoporotic fractures since the risk of falling is increased due to various factors such as poor vision, muscle weakness and postural instability. The most important risk factors include:

- Family history
- Early menopause
- Low body weight
- Poor diet
- Drug treatments:
  - Corticosteroids
  - Aromatase inhibitors
  - GnRH agonists
- Coexisting disease:
  - RA and other chronic inflammatory diseases
  - Malabsorption
  - Chronic liver and kidney diseases
  - Thyrotoxicosis, hyperparathyroidism and other endocrine diseases.

Presentation

Low BMD does not cause symptoms and typically the clinical presentation is with a fracture. Fractures can affect any bone, but the three most common sites are the wrist, hip and spine. A fracture is associated with a greatly increased risk of subsequent fractures. Clinical signs include:

- Height loss, kyphosis and back pain (vertebral fracture)
- Painful, shortened and externally rotated hip (hip fracture)
- Pain and deformity of affected bone (other fractures).

Investigations

- Routine bloods: often normal. Hypercalcaemia in primary hyperparathyroidism; abnormal LFT or U&E in chronic liver or kidney disease; low testosterone in male hypogonadism; raised ESR and paraprotein in multiple myeloma; paraprotein in monoclonal gammopathy of uncertain significance; raised T4 and low thyroid stimulating hormone (TSH) in thyrotoxicosis
- Immunology: raised tissue transglutaminase (TTG) in occult coeliac disease
- Imaging: radiographs may show evidence of fracture or wedge deformity of vertebrae. The diagnosis is made by DEXA which in osteoporotic individuals

TABLE 5.6	
BONE DENSITY THRESHOLDS FOR INITIATION OF DRUG TREATMENT OF OSTEOPOROSIS	
Patient Group	**Treatment Threshold (T-Score)**
Postmenopausal osteoporosis	−2.5
Osteoporosis in men aged >50	−2.5
Corticosteroid-induced osteoporosis	−1.5

shows a T-score <−2.5 at spine or hip (see Chapter 3). Note that osteoporosis may be present with normal spine BMD in patients with vertebral fracture, due to coexisting OA or aortic calcification.

Management
The aims of management are to prevent fractures. Pharmacological and nonpharmacological approaches are both important. The T-score on DEXA scanning can be used to guide the need for treatment (Table 5.6).

CORE DRUG TREATMENTS
- Alendronic acid or risedronate first choices
- Zoledronic acid if oral drugs contraindicated or for GI intolerance
- Denosumab if zoledronic acid contraindicated or in patients with poor renal function
- Teriparatide for severe spinal osteoporosis
- Calcium and vitamin D supplements mainly as adjunct to other treatments.

OTHER TREATMENT OPTIONS
- HRT – early menopause, women <60 years if age
- Raloxifene – younger women with spinal osteoporosis
- Tibolone – younger women with spinal osteoporosis
- Ibandronate – limited role as alternative other bisphosphonates (nonvertebral fracture data limited)
- Strontium ranelate – only to be used in severe osteoporosis, if other drugs are unsuitable and no evidence of (or risk factors for) cardiovascular disease.

NONPHARMACOLOGICAL
- Maintain good diet with adequate calcium and vitamin D
- Stop smoking
- Reduce alcohol below 21 units/week for men and 14 for women
- Assess falls risk and introduce prevention strategies if appropriate.

  HINTS AND TIPS

OSTEOPOROSIS

Fracture risk assessments with QFracture or FRAX are now used to prioritize patients for DEXA examination, although DEXA is also offered in many centres (through fracture liaison services) to all patients over 50 years of age who suffer a fracture. Elderly patients with spinal osteoporosis may have a false negative result on DEXA examination due to artefacts such as aortic calcification and degenerative disease of the spine.

OSTEOMALACIA AND RICKETS

 OVERVIEW

Osteomalacia is characterized by impaired mineralization of bone and the accumulation of thickened seams of uncalcified bone (osteoid) on bone surfaces. When this occurs in the growing skeleton it is known as rickets and results in bone deformity and growth retardation. The aims of management are to improve symptoms and to restore normal biochemistry.

The most common cause of osteomalacia is vitamin D deficiency but it can occur as the result of various genetic disorders that cause renal phosphate wasting or affect the molecular mechanisms of vitamin D action or metabolism. Muslim women and elderly housebound individuals are at increased risk since vitamin D is mostly derived from exposure to sunlight.

Pathogenesis

Vitamin D can be derived from the diet (mainly oily fish) or by the action of ultraviolet light on the skin that converts 7-dehydrocholesterol to cholecalciferol (vitamin D). Thereafter the vitamin D undergoes hydroxylation in the liver at the 25-position to yield 25(OH)D and further hydroxylation at the 1-position to give the active metabolite $1,25(OH)_2D_3$ (Figure 5.9). The resulting $1,25(OH)_2D_3$ promotes calcium and phosphate absorption from the gut and promotes osteoclastic bone resorption. In the presence of vitamin D deficiency, intestinal absorption of calcium (and phosphate) is reduced causing serum calcium levels to fall. This is detected by the parathyroid glands that secrete PTH and increase bone turnover, which releases calcium from bone into the circulation but causes phosphaturia and hypophosphataemia. If vitamin D deficiency is severe and prolonged there is progressive demineralization of bone due to a sustained elevation in PTH (secondary hyperparathyroidism) leading eventually to osteomalacia or rickets. Less common causes of osteomalacia and rickets include:

- Inherited mutations in the genes that regulate vitamin D metabolism (vitamin D–resistant rickets)
- Inherited mutations in genes that regulate phosphate metabolism (hypophosphataemic rickets)
- Acquired defects in phosphate metabolism (tumour-induced osteomalacia)
- Chronic renal failure (failure of $1,25(OH)_2D_3$ synthesis by the kidneys)
- Bisphosphonates, and aluminum toxicity.

Presentation

The presenting features of osteomalacia include:

- Bone pain and/or tenderness
- Muscle weakness and fatigue
- General malaise
- Fracture.

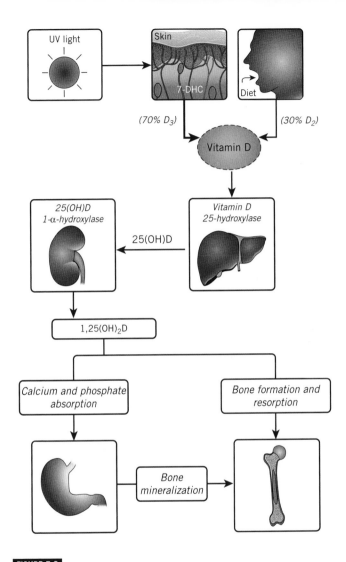

FIGURE 5.9

Vitamin D metabolism. Circulating vitamin D made in the skin by the action of UV light on 7-dehydrocholesterol (vitamin D3) and also obtained from the diet (vitamin D2). It has been estimated that skin synthesis accounts for about 70% of vitamin D levels in most people. Circulating vitamin D is hydroxylated by the liver to form 25(OH)D and is further hydroxylated by the kidney to form the active metabolite $1,25(OH)_2D_3$. The $1,25(OH)_2D_3$ increased absorption of calcium and phosphate absorption from the gut and this in turn promotes bone mineralization. Vitamin D also has direct effects on bone formation and resorption by regulating osteoblasts and osteoclast differentiation.

The presenting features of rickets include:

- Bone pain and deformity
- Bone expansion at the epiphyseal plate
- Delayed development and failure to thrive
- Tetany and seizures.

Investigations

- Routine bloods: calcium normal or low/normal; hypophosphataemia, raised PTH, 25(OH) undetectable, alkaline phosphatase raised
- Imaging: osteopenia on X-ray with fractures or pseudofractures (Figure 5.10); widened epiphyses in children
- Bone biopsy: seldom necessary but shows increased bone turnover with increased thickness and extent of osteoid seams.

Management

The approach to treatment depends on the underlying cause.

OSTEOMALACIA CAUSED BY VITAMIN D DEFICIENCY

This responds rapidly and completely to cholecalciferol. Traditionally, high doses of vitamin D have been used but osteomalacia can also be successfully treated by moderate doses of cholecalciferol such as 2400–3200 units daily (100 μg/day) for 1–2 months. In the UK licensed preparations are available providing 400 (12.5 μg), 800 (25 μg) and 25 000 units of vitamin D (625 μg). The dose and duration of therapy should be tailored to the clinical response and response of ALP levels (ALP levels fall to normal when osteomalacia is healed). Patients should be continued on a maintenance dose of 800–1600 units daily to prevent recurrence.

HYPOPHOSPHATAEMIA RICKETS

Active vitamin D metabolites (Alfacalcidol 1–3 μg daily or Rocaltrol 0.5–2 μg daily) plus phosphate supplements. The dose and duration of therapy should be tailored to the clinical response and response of ALP and serum phosphate levels (ALP levels fall to normal when osteomalacia is healed).

CHRONIC RENAL FAILURE

Active vitamin D metabolites (Alfacalcidol 1–3 μg daily or Rocaltrol 0.5–2 μg daily) with adjustment of the dose according to clinical response and response of ALP and serum calcium levels.

PAGET DISEASE

 OVERVIEW

Paget disease of bone is characterized by focal increases in bone remodelling, which result in the production of abnormal bone that is mechanically weak. Bone pain is the most common presenting often in association with raised ALP levels and typical x-ray findings. The aim of management is to control pain. There is no evidence, as yet, that treatment can reduce the risk of complications.

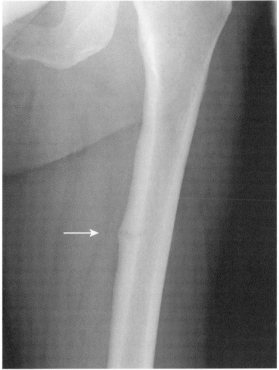

A radiograph of the left femur in a patient with osteomalacia, demonstrating a pseudofracture in the medial cortex. The patient was housebound with a poor diet and presented with bone pain and muscle weakness.

The bones most commonly involved in Paget disease include the pelvis, spine, skull, femur and tibia. It is rare under the age of 50 but the prevalence doubles each decade thereafter to affect about 8% of the UK population over the age of 80. It is more common in men (1.4:1). There are also marked ethnic differences in susceptibility: the disease is common in the UK and other parts of Europe (except Scandinavia), but is extremely rare in the Far East and the Indian subcontinent.

Pathogenesis

Genetic factors play an important role. The most important gene is *SQSTM1*; mutations are found in about 40–50% of patients with a family history and about 10% of patients overall. The disease-causing mutations increase osteoclast activity, and several other genes and susceptibility loci have been identified. Environmental factors also contribute and suggested triggers for the

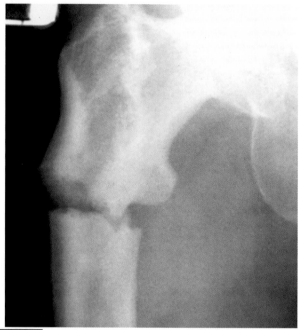

Pathological fracture associated with Paget disease.

disease include a poor diet, exposure to infections, skeletal damage and repetitive mechanical loading.

Presentation

Many patients are asymptomatic and it has been estimated that only 7–15% come to medical attention. In those that do, the most common presenting features are:

- Bone pain
- Bone deformity
- Pathological fracture (Figure 5.11)
- Increased temperature over an affected bone
- Hearing loss
- Joint pain due to OA
- Spinal stenosis.

Rare complications include:

- Hypercalcaemia (with immobilization)
- High-output cardiac failure (increased blood flow through bone)

- Hydrocephalus (due to skull involvement)
- Osteosarcoma.

Investigations

- Routine bloods: raised ALP with other bloods often normal
- Imaging: abnormal trabecular pattern with alternating osteosclerosis and osteolysis; bone expansion and deformity, and pseudofractures. Homogenous increase of tracer uptake in affected bones
- Bone biopsy: seldom required, classically shows increased osteoclast and osteoblast activity; marrow fibrosis and woven bone.

Management

The primary aim of therapy is to improve bone pain, which can be achieved by antiresorptive drugs if the pain is thought to be due to increased bone turnover or by analgesics and NSAIDs. The response to antiresorptive treatment can be followed biochemically by measuring ALP levels. Although antiresorptive drugs can help pain, there is no evidence as yet to show that they can prevent complications such as fractures or deformity.

Drug Treatment

- Risedronate 30 mg daily orally for 2 months
- Zoledronic acid 5 mg i.v. once
- Pamidronate 60 mg i.v. on three occasions
- Etidronate and tiludronate 400 mg daily for 3–6 months (seldom used)
- Calcitonin 100 i.u. 3 times/week (if other drugs contraindicated)
- Analgesics/NSAIDs for pain.

Further courses of bisphosphonates can be given for recurrence of pain if it is thought to be due to reactivation of the disease and accompanied by an elevation in ALP.

Nonpharmacological Treatment

- Shoe raises (deformity due to limb shortening)
- Walking aids.

Surgery

- Fracture fixation
- Joint replacement (secondary OA)
- Spinal stenosis
- Osteotomy for deformity
- Osteosarcoma (prognosis poor even with amputation).

 HINTS AND TIPS

PAGET DISEASE

Long bone bowing are classical features on radiographs of the femur or tibia. Joint replacement surgery can be technically difficult due to an increased risk of bleeding, as well as bone deformity making alignment difficult. Osteosarcoma is an uncommon complication occurring in less than 0.1% of patients, but has a very poor 5-year survival rate even with aggressive treatment.

FIBROUS DYSPLASIA

 OVERVIEW

Fibrous dysplasia is characterized by bone pain, pathological fracture and, occasionally, deformity of the bone due to focal or multifocal osteolytic lesions. The aims of management are to improve symptoms and treat endocrine disease, if present.

Fibrous dysplasia may affect a single bone (monostotic) or multiple bones (polyostotic). Polyostotic fibrous dysplasia may be associated with café-au-lait skin pigmentation, precocious puberty and other endocrine abnormalities, and this is referred to as McCune–Albright syndrome.

Pathogenesis

The cause is a gain-of-function somatic mutation in the Gs-alpha protein that is responsible for signal transduction downstream of various G-protein coupled receptors (GPCR). The causal mutations mimic the effects of hormone activation. The mutations are not inherited in the germ line but instead occur in somatic cells during early embryonic development; as a result, the daughter cells carrying the mutations can occur throughout the body, but in a patchy distribution. The effects of the mutations are predominantly seen in bone and the endocrine system because the effects of many endocrine hormones are mediated by binding to G-protein-coupled receptors.

Presentation

- Bone pain
- Pathological fracture
- Bone deformity
- Precocious puberty
- Café-au-lait pigmentation
- Hypophosphataemic rickets (rare)
- Thyrotoxicosis, Cushing syndrome and acromegaly (rare)
- Sarcoma in affected bones (rare).

Investigations

- Routine bloods: normal
- Imaging: focal osteolytic lesions and bone expansion. Osteosclerosis less prominent. Local increase in tracer uptake on isotope bone scan; and bone marrow oedema on MRI
- Bone biopsy: seldom required but shows increased osteoclast numbers and activity, marrow fibrosis, and increased bone formation less prominent than with Paget disease.

Management

Includes:

- Intravenous bisphosphonates for bone pain (evidence base weak):
  - Pamidronate 60 mg intravenous every 3–6 months
- Analgesics and NSAIDs for bone pain

- Phosphate supplements and vitamin D metabolites for hypophosphataemic rickets
- Orthopaedic surgery for fracture fixation and bone deformity
- Aromatase inhibitors may be used for precocious puberty in females and antiandrogens in males
- Thyrotoxicosis, Cushing syndrome and acromegaly may require specific treatment.

Prognosis

The prognosis is generally good with a normal life expectancy but some patients may suffer morbidity associated with pathological fractures, deformity and endocrinopathy.

Chapter 6

Regional Orthopaedics and Trauma

CHAPTER OUTLINE

SHOULDER AND ARM
ELBOW AND FOREARM
WRIST AND HAND
PELVIS, HIP AND KNEE
   Hip and Knee Arthroplasty
ANKLE AND FOOT

HEAD, NECK AND SPINE
BONE AND JOINT INFECTIONS
MUSCULOSKELETAL TUMOURS
NERVE INJURIES

Fracture classification, general initial assessment and management, and general complications are discussed in Chapter 4.

SHOULDER AND ARM

Clavicle Fractures

A clavicular fracture often occurs at the point between the middle and distal thirds, with inferior displacement of the distal fracture fragment due to the effect of gravity on the arm, whereas the sternomastoid muscle displaces the proximal fragment superiorly.

Presentation

- Common in young males
- Direct fall onto the shoulder or FOOSH
- Shoulder and clavicular region pain and tenderness
- Visible protrusion along clavicular line:
  - Skin tenting and open fracture possible
- Essential to assess the distal neurovascular status:
  - Brachial plexus, subclavian vessels, axillary nerve and artery.

Investigations

- Clavicle AP radiograph and 30° caudal:
  - Position and deformity (Figure 6.1).

Management

- Conservative:
  - Immobilization (sling or collar and cuff) is usually sufficient
- Surgical:
  - Open reduction and internal fixation (screws and plate, intramedullary rods)

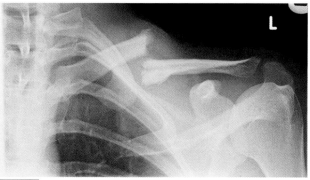

Displaced fracture of the midshaft of the left clavicle.

- Relative indications include displaced lateral fractures, shortening of the clavicle, open fractures, soft tissue (neurovascular) compromise, bilateral fractures and multiple trauma, e.g. flail chest and symptomatic nonunions.

Complications

- Postoperative:
  - Infection
  - Removal of metalwork
  - Neurovascular injury
- Malunion (impinged shoulder abduction) or nonunion (~5–10%):
  - Higher rate with lateral fractures
- Brachial plexus injury (high energy)
- Pneumothorax (high energy).

Anterior Glenohumeral Dislocation

 OVERVIEW

Glenohumeral joint dislocation is one of the commonest dislocations as it is a shallow and intrinsically unstable joint. It is commonly anterior and traumatic, requiring early reduction in the emergency department or in theatre if this is not possible. It is essential to assess for an associated fracture around the shoulder, as well as the neurovascular status of the affected limb. After reduction most patients can be managed nonoperatively in a sling with early physiotherapy. Beware: elderly patients have a high rate of associated rotator cuff tears, while young and active patients have a high rate of recurrence. The *terrible triad* shoulder dislocation is a dislocation with associated rotator cuff tear and axillary nerve injury.

The stability of the shoulder joint is maintained by the glenoid labrum and the capsule, ligaments and rotator cuff muscles, which hold the humeral head against the flat glenoid. The mechanism of an anterior shoulder dislocation is often traumatic (a fall backwards onto an outstretched hand, i.e. when the shoulder is forced into abduction and external rotation) with head displacement in the anterior–inferior direction (~95%). The forward displacement of the humeral head often leads to injury of the labrum and anterior capsule.

Presentation

- Shoulder pain with a restricted (often no) range of movement
- Affected fixed arm supported by opposite arm or held by side
- Gross deformity: regular lateral contour lost (more a square shape on presentation) with a palpable step and bulge (humeral head)
- Assess neurovascular status:
  - Axillary nerve.

Investigations

- Shoulder radiograph (AP and axillary or 'Y' views):
  - Humeral head will often be visible medially and inferiorly to the glenoid (Figure 6.2)
  - Coexisting proximal humeral fracture (greater tuberosity)
- CT or MRI:
  - Define associated bony and/or soft tissue injury.

Management

- Conservative:
  - Immediate reduction with analgesia and sedation using Kocher (traction, external rotation, adduction, internal rotation), Milch or the Hippocratic method is the norm

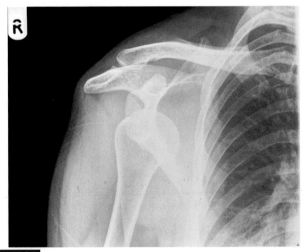

FIGURE 6.2
Anterior dislocation of the right shoulder joint.

- Check radiograph post-reduction
- Immobilization (e.g. collar and cuff) and early physiotherapy
- Surgical:
  - Arthroscopic exploration and stabilization offered depending on associated lesion(s), age and activities.

Complications

- Postreduction:
  - Axillary nerve damage or humeral head fracture
- Recurrent dislocation:
  - 80% due to damage of the labrum and capsule (as discussed later); younger age most important predictor for recurrence
- Rotator cuff tear (e.g. subscapularis) and stiffness:
  - Elderly
- Neurovascular injury:
  - Axillary nerve neurapraxia ('regimental patch sign')
  - Brachial plexus damage also possible.

 PROCEDURE

REDUCTION OF A SHOULDER DISLOCATION

INDICATIONS

- Closed reduction for simple dislocations, or those associated with tuberosity fractures
- More complex fracture-dislocations may require open reduction and internal fixation, and discussion with a senior colleague prior to reduction is recommended

CONSENT

- Risk of neurovascular injury
- Risk of iatrogenic fracture
- Risk of failure necessitating an open reduction

PROCEDURE

The patient is placed supine. Successful reduction relies upon adequate muscle relaxation rather than excessive force, and can be achieved potentially in the conscious patient with analgesia and the slow application of traction, or with the aid of systemic sedation or anaesthesia. Methods of closed reduction include:

- Hippocratic:
  - Longitudinal traction is applied to the extended arm
  - Countertraction is applied to the chest using a sheet around the body, with care to avoid pressure in the axilla
  - Alternatively and traditionally, a foot (without shoe) placed on the chest wall, and the ball of the foot is used as a fulcrum to manoeuvre the humeral head laterally whilst supplying traction and adduction to the arm
  - Slight external rotation of the arm may help disengage the humeral head from its position on the glenoid rim
- Milch:
  - Apply longitudinal traction to the arm in the neutral position
  - Whilst maintaining traction apply gradual abduction whilst controlling rotation of the humeral head

PROCEDURE—cont'd

- Kocher:
  - Flex the elbow to 90° with the arm in neutral abduction and apply longitudinal traction
  - Slowly externally rotate the arm to 90°, using the forearm as a lever
  - The arm is then adducted across the chest and then internally rotated (to bring the hand to the contralateral shoulder)
  - This manoeuvre should be used with caution in elderly or osteoporotic individuals due to the risk of humeral head fractures

  Post-manipulation the shoulder is immobilized in a sling. A postreduction check radiograph is essential to ensure the shoulder is reduced and there is no associated fracture, along with a repeat assessment of the neurovascular status of the limb.

Posterior Glenohumeral Dislocation

Posterior dislocations are rare and are associated with seizure (epileptics), electrocution or a direct blow to the anterior aspect of the shoulder that forces the arm into abduction and internal rotation, with head displacement in the posteroinferior direction. The diagnosis can be missed.

Presentation
- Intense shoulder pain with no range of movement
- Arm held in internal rotation (loss of external rotation).

Investigations
- Shoulder radiograph (AP and axillary or 'Y' views):
  - AP is often normal apart from the 'light bulb sign' (Figure 6.3)
  - Confirm with axillary/lateral view
- CT or MRI.

Management
- Immediate reduction (often under GA) using closed (traction and external rotation) or open method
- Immobilization and early physiotherapy
- Same as anterior treatment thereafter.

Recurrent Glenohumeral Dislocation

Recurrent dislocation often follows an anterior dislocation and is normally due to the following factors, the first two of which are a consequence of the first dislocation and reduce the stable arc of glenohumeral motion, although younger age is the strongest predictor:

- Posterolateral indentation fracture of the humeral head (Hill–Sachs lesion, see Figure 6.3)
- Capsule and labrum damage at the anterior joint margin (Bankart lesion)
- Younger age (strong risk factor for recurrent dislocation)
- Elderly with rotator cuff disease
- Atraumatic, e.g. Ehlers–Danlos syndrome
- Habitual.

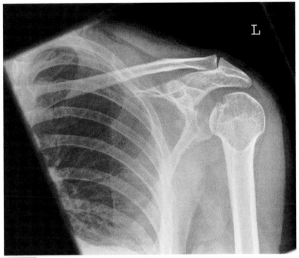

FIGURE 6.3

The 'light bulb sign' is clear with a rotated humeral head in the AP view. A reverse Hill–Sachs lesion is visible on the surface of the humeral head and a CT scan will help define such a lesion.

Presentation

- As in primary dislocation:
  - Can have minimal pain
- Positive anterior (patient supine so scapula supported but shoulder/arm free, arm in 90 degrees abduction and external rotation, controlled anterior force) or posterior (patient supine so scapula supported but arm free, arm in adduction and flexion, controlled posterior force on proximal humerus) apprehension test.

Investigations

- Shoulder radiograph (AP and axillary or 'Y' views):
- CT or MRI.

Management

- Conservative:
  - Self-reduction sometimes possible
  - Immobilization and early physiotherapy
- Surgical:
  - Anterior capsule reconstruction for anterior dislocation (Bankart, Putti–Platt, inferior capsular shift operations)
  - Recurrent posterior dislocation requires bone and soft tissue reconstruction
  - Habitual or multidirectional instability should be treated conservatively.

Dislocation of the Sternoclavicular or Acromioclavicular Joints

Injuries to the sternoclavicular and acromioclavicular (Rockwood classification) joints are rare but when they do occur they often involve subluxation or dislocation of the joint surface. These can often be treated with a broad arm sling, providing there is no neurovascular compromise and limited displacement. OA is a potential complication. Posterior sternoclavicular joint dislocation can cause damage to the mediastinal structures and requires potentially urgent joint orthopaedic and cardiothoracic assessment.

Fractures of the Humerus

See Table 6.1.

TABLE 6.1

THE SUBTYPES, PRESENTATION AND MANAGEMENT OF HUMERAL FRACTURES

Subtype	Presentation and Investigations	Management (Complications)
Proximal: • Humeral head • Greater tuberosity • Lesser tuberosity • Surgical neck	Elderly, osteoporosis Fall onto shoulder/arm (direct blow) or FOOSH Assess for deformity, bruising (haemarthrosis), rotator cuff, dislocation, axillary nerve and vascular status Radiographs (Neer classification) CT may be required	Analgesia Minimal/moderate displacement: sling immobilization Severe displacement/head-splitting/fracture dislocation: surgery considered, e.g. reduction and internal fixation, hemi-arthroplasty* (Axillary nerve/artery injury, skin compromise, brachial plexus injury, stiffness, dislocation, malunion, nonunion, avascular necrosis of humeral head)
Shaft	Elderly, FOOSH, twisting mechanism Assess for deformity, radial nerve and distal vascular status Radiographs	Analgesia Minimal/moderate displacement: U-slab then bracing Severe displacement/unstable: surgery considered, e.g. ORIF with a plate (Radial nerve injury pre- and postop, nonunion)
Distal	Elderly, FOOSH, high energy in young Assess for deformity, open injury, neurovascular status Radiographs +/– CT	Analgesia Majority managed with ORIF unless undisplaced Nonoperative (bag of bones technique) is used by some for elderly lower demand patients

*AP, lateral/axial views are required for thorough assessment of the proximal humerus. Displacement of the proximal humerus is traditionally defined as a significant fragment that is angulated >45° and/or displaced >1 cm. It is important to assess the patient's normal functional demands when considering surgical options.

HINTS AND TIPS

SHOULDER AND ARM TRAUMA

It is essential to assess the neurovascular status of the affected limb following an injury to the shoulder, particularly before and after any reduction of a dislocated shoulder and when assessing a humeral shaft fracture. For a dislocation of the

HINTS AND TIPS—cont'd

shoulder, assess axillary nerve (regimental badge sign and deltoid function) and artery status (palpate brachial or radial artery). For a fracture of the humeral shaft it is important to assess radial nerve function (wrist and finger extension, and sensation first dorsal web space) before and after immobilization. 85–90% of radial nerve palsy presenting concomitantly with a humeral shaft fracture will resolve spontaneously.

Rotator Cuff Disease

 OVERVIEW

Rotator cuff disease (which commonly involves supraspinatus) presents due to inflammation, degeneration, injury or a revascularization/calcium deposition reaction. Ultrasound and/or MRI are diagnostic and treatment is dependent on the patient, any tear characteristics and the associated disability.

A sheet of joined tendons that make up the rotator cuff covers the shoulder capsule and inserts into the greater and lesser tuberosities of the humerus. The muscles of the rotator cuff are:

- Supraspinatus (abduction)
- Subscapularis (internal rotation)
- Infraspinatus (external rotation)
- Teres minor (external rotation and adduction).

The stability of the glenohumeral joint is determined by the functionality of these muscles and the sheet of tendons associated with them. Rotator cuff disease, a degeneration of these tendons – in particular the avascular region near the insertion of the supraspinatus tendon – is commonly seen after 40 years of age, and can lead to a partial or complete tear of the tendon(s). Common causes are:

- Rotator cuff tears as a result of trauma or chronic impingement between the acromion and greater tuberosity:
  - Acute on chronic tear
- Calcific tendinitis
- Impingement of cuff.

Presentation (Table 6.2)

- Dependent on tendon(s) involved and the underlying cause
- Impingement is characterized by a painful arc
- A tear can be associated with a painless loss of function
- See Chapter 2 for assessment of the cuff:
  - Special tests include Neer, Hawkins and Jobe test.

Investigations

- Radiographs:
  - Tears: degenerative changes and high riding humerus
  - Impingement: subacromial sclerosis
  - Calcific tendinitis: calcific deposit

TABLE 6.2

THE SUBTYPES, PRESENTATION AND MANAGEMENT OF ROTATOR CUFF DISEASE*

Subtype	Presentation and Investigations	Management (Complications)
Rotator cuff impingement	Middle-aged Good range of passive movement Painful arc test positive (~60–120°)	Physiotherapy and NSAIDs Subacromial steroid injection – can be diagnostic Subacromial decompression (Recurrence)
Rotator cuff tear	Middle-aged or elderly Painless loss of function Possible history of trauma Identify affected muscle using tests described in Chapter 2 Confirm on ultrasound +/– MRI	Individualized to age, functional demand and type of tear (Recurrence post surgical repair)
Calcific tendonitis	Middle-aged (20–50 years) Associated with diabetes Often no history of trauma Rapid onset of severe pain and loss of function Impingement may be seen Shoulder radiograph: calcific deposit within supraspinatus tendon	Rest and NSAIDs Steroid injection +/– US guided barbotage Subacromial deposit removal (Recurrence)

*Subacromial bursitis is seen as an early stage of rotator cuff tendonitis (impingement). For how to assess the muscles of the rotator cuff, please see Chapter 2.

Adapted from Frost A, Robinson CM. The painful shoulder. Surgery 2006; 24(11): 363–367.

- USS:
  - Concomitant injection for suspected impingement +/– barbotage for calcific deposit
- MRI or MR-arthrogram.

Management (Table 6.2)

- Conservative:
  - Immobilization (e.g. collar and cuff) best avoided
  - Physiotherapy
  - Corticosteroid injection of subacromial bursa (improved symptoms can be diagnostic for impingement)
- Surgical:
  - Arthroscopic subacromial decompression and debridement
  - Arthroscopic removal of calcific deposit in recalcitrant cases
  - Arthroscopic or open rotator cuff repair (for complete symptomatic tears in active patients).

Frozen Shoulder

Adhesive capsulitis or frozen shoulder is a common idiopathic condition of the shoulder that may also occurs after minor trauma or recent surgery to the shoulder or upper limb, where there has been a period of immobility. Patients are characteristically middle aged (with women in the sixth decade being the most common), and may have a background of diabetes, IHD or thyroid disease.

Presentation

- Spontaneous onset of a painful and stiff shoulder
- Global reduction in shoulder movement:
  - Limited active and passive
  - Pathognomonic loss of external rotation.

Investigations

- Radiographs:
  - Exclude concomitant rotator cuff disease but often normal
- MRI +/– arthrogram.

Management

- Conservative:
  - Effective in many cases but can take 1–3 years to resolve
  - Physiotherapy and NSAIDs
  - Steroid injection
  - Distension arthrogram with immediate physiotherapy.
- Surgical:
  - For refractory cases
  - MUA (manipulation under anaesthesia)
  - Arthroscopic release +/– decompression.

 HINTS AND TIPS

ROTATOR CUFF DISEASE

Supraspinatus is responsible for initiation of glenohumeral abduction, so a rotator cuff tear that commonly involves supraspinatus, will affect this action. However, limited active abduction is also possible due to scapular-thoracic rotation and deltoid abduction. An important prerequisite of total shoulder arthroplasty for shoulder arthritis is an intact rotator cuff.

ELBOW AND FOREARM

Elbow Dislocation

 OVERVIEW

A dislocation of the elbow commonly occurs following a fall onto an outstretched hand with the elbow in flexion. Pre- and postreduction radiographs need to be scrutinized for concomitant fractures to the proximal forearm or distal humerus. Management is often conservative for an isolated dislocation. For fracture-dislocations of the elbow, instability is possible and surgery may be required.

An elbow dislocation is commonly characterized by a posterior displacement (most common form, with anterior and medial/lateral less common) of the proximal ulna relative to the distal humerus.

Presentation

- Elbow pain and swelling with a restricted range of movement

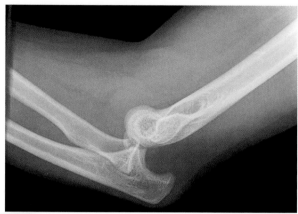

FIGURE 6.4

Posterior dislocation of the elbow.

- Gross deformity often apparent:
  - Elbow triangle symmetry lost (olecranon and condyles) with olecranon prominent
  - Elbow held in flexion by other arm
- It is essential to assess the neurovascular status of the affected limb before and after reduction:
  - In particular, assess median/ulnar nerve and distal vascular status.

Investigations

- Elbow radiograph (AP and lateral)
- CT for complex fracture-dislocations:
  - Position of dislocation (Figure 6.4)
  - Coexisting fracture(s) possible, e.g. radial head, coronoid process and proximal ulna.

Management

- Conservative:
  - Immediate reduction with analgesia and sedation, with check radiograph postreduction
  - Immobilization (e.g. above-elbow back slab with elbow at 90°) for a maximum of 2 weeks to avoid long-term stiffness
- Surgical:
  - Considered for fracture-dislocations with instability, e.g. terrible triad injury (posterior dislocation of elbow, radial head fracture, coronoid fracture)
  - Internal fixation of significant intraarticular or unstable fractures, ligament repair (often lateral collateral) +/– radial head replacement.

Complications

- Instability:
  - Persistent early instability can be treated with targeted elbow exercises and/or a hinged external fixator depending on severity
- Stiffness, pain and/or delayed recovery of function:
  - Increased with complex fracture-dislocations
  - HO (heterotopic ossification) or myositis ossicans
  - OA
- Neurovascular injury:
  - Median, radial and/or ulnar nerve neurapraxia
  - Brachial artery (rare)
- Recurrent dislocation (rare)
- Postreduction:
  - Neurovascular injury.

Olecranon Fractures

These fractures are commonly seen as the result of direct trauma (e.g. a fall onto the elbow) and occur both in younger patients following a high-energy fall, as well as in older patients with a low-energy fall.

Presentation

- Pain and swelling over posterior aspect of elbow
- Reduced range of movement:
  - Inability to fully extend the elbow
  - Palpable gap can sometimes be felt
- Assess carefully for an open injury.

Investigation

- Elbow radiograph (AP and lateral):
  - Mayo classification commonly used (three types based upon displacement, elbow instability and fracture comminution).

Management

- Conservative:
  - Undisplaced fractures (<2 mm articular surface)
  - Displaced fractures in elderly lower demand patients
  - Collar and cuff or above elbow plaster immobilization
- Surgical:
  - Displaced and/or unstable fractures
  - Tension band wire fixation most commonly used for simple transverse fractures
  - Plate fixation used for comminuted, distal, oblique and unstable patterns.

Complications

- Postsurgery:
  - Symptomatic hardware (high removal rate)
  - HO
  - Neurovascular injury
- Pain and stiffness

- Loss of extension strength
- Secondary OA.

Radial Head Fractures

A fracture of the radial head is the most common fracture occurring around the elbow and is usually seen following a FOOSH. Radial neck fractures are most frequently seen in children.

Presentation

- Pain and swelling over lateral aspect of the elbow
- Inability to fully extend the elbow:
  - Assess forearm pronation and supination.
- Varus–valgus instability if possible
- Important to consider concomitant osseous and ligamentous injuries:
  - Proximal ulna/coronoid/distal humerus fractures
  - Elbow dislocation +/– terrible triad injury
  - Essex-Lopresti injury
  - Carpal fractures.

Investigation

- Elbow radiograph (AP and lateral):
  - Haemarthrosis may cause a positive fat pad sign
  - Mason classification (types 1–3).

Management

- Conservative:
  - The vast majority of isolated type 1 and type 2 fractures
  - Brief immobilization with collar and cuff
  - Some advocate joint aspiration +/– injection of LA
  - Early active motion +/– physiotherapy
- Surgical:
  - Only absolute indication is a true block to forearm rotation
  - Role of ORIF in Mason type 2 fractures debated but no advantage proven
  - Considered for complex displaced fractures associated with instability of the elbow and/or forearm, e.g. terrible triad injury
  - Radial head replacement used when ORIF not possible (common) and instability suspected
  - Acute radial head excision for comminuted fractures not associated with elbow/forearm instability (rare)
  - Delayed radial head excision for ongoing pain and stiffness.

Complications

- Postsurgery:
  - Posterior interosseous nerve injury
  - Loss of fixation
  - Infection
- Instability
- Pain and stiffness
- Secondary OA.

Forearm Fractures

These fractures are commonly seen as a result of either direct or indirect trauma. One bone (e.g. isolated ulnar shaft fracture – nightstick injury), both bones, or one bone and the elbow or wrist joint can be involved. Any displaced fracture of the forearm can result in disturbance of forearm rotation, with anatomical reduction and fixation recommended.

Presentation
- Pain, swelling and deformity to the forearm
- It is essential to assess the neurovascular status of the affected limb
- Careful assessment for an open fracture.

Investigations
- Forearm radiographs (AP and lateral):
  - Should include elbow and wrist joint with focused views of joint(s) as required.

Management
- Conservative:
  - For an undisplaced or minimally displaced isolated single bone diaphyseal fracture of the ulna, i.e. nightstick fracture
  - Immobilization (e.g. above-elbow back slab with elbow at 90°)
- Surgical:
  - ORIF is preferred treatment in most cases
  - Important to assess supination and pronation intraoperatively.

Complications
- Compartment syndrome (rare)
- Infection postoperatively
- Nonunion or malunion (rare with good fixation)
- Neurovascular injury (e.g. radial or posterior interosseous nerve)
- Pain and stiffness
- Re-fracture
- Removal of metalwork
- Synostosis in severe injury or if both bones fixed through a single incision.

 HINTS AND TIPS

ELBOW AND FOREARM TRAUMA

It is essential that both the elbow and wrist are x-rayed at presentation, particularly if there are any concomitant symptoms and/or signs. Distal occult fractures or soft tissue injuries can occur. Examples include:

1. Monteggia fracture-dislocation where there is a fracture of the ulna (often proximal) with an associated dislocation of the radial head.
2. Galeazzi fracture-dislocation where there is a fracture of the radius (often shaft) and a distal radial ulnar joint dislocation.
3. Essex-Lopresti type injury with a fracture of the proximal radius and an associated injury of the interosseous membrane and disruption of the distal radial ulnar joint leading to radial shortening.

Tennis Elbow

Tennis elbow, or lateral epicondylitis, is the chronic inflammation, degeneration and rupture of aponeurotic fibres of the common extensor tendon (often extensor carpi radialis brevis) where it originates from the lateral supracondylar ridge of the humerus. It is commonly caused by eccentric loading secondary to minor trauma or repetitive strain, occurring when the extensors of the arm are contracted, accompanied by sharp flexion of the wrist, e.g. a backhand stroke in tennis.

Presentation

- Pain and tenderness at the humeral lateral epicondyle/common extensor origin
- Reproducible pain on resisted wrist or finger extension
- Normal flexion and extension of the elbow
- Grip strength can be reduced secondary to pain.

Management

- Conservative:
  - Effective for majority
  - Activity modification +/− bracing
  - Analgesia, e.g. NSAIDs and physiotherapy
  - Corticosteroid injection (efficacy debated)
- Surgical:
  - Rarely indicated
  - Common extensor origin debridement and release.

Golfer's Elbow

Golfer's elbow, or medial epicondylitis, is the chronic inflammation, degeneration and rupture of aponeurotic fibres of the common flexor tendon (commonly pronator teres and flexor carpi radialis) where it originates from the medial supracondylar ridge of the humerus. Pain is commonly caused by strain occurring with hyperextension of the wrist and fingers, e.g. a golfer striking the ground, not the ball. It is less common than tennis elbow.

Presentation

- Pain at the medial condyle, tender to touch
- Tenderness area less precise than with tennis elbow
- Normal flexion and extension of the elbow
- Reproducible pain on resisted wrist flexion.

Management

- Conservative:
  - Analgesia and physiotherapy
  - Corticosteroid injection (efficacy debated)
- Surgical:
  - Rarely indicated
  - Common flexor origin stripping and release.

HINTS AND TIPS

TENNIS AND GOLFER'S ELBOW

The 't' in lateral is used to remember that tennis elbow is lateral epicondylitis. Although there are advocates for local corticosteroid injection, there is substantial evidence to suggest this does not aid with the resolution of symptoms.

Olecranon Bursitis

Olecranon bursitis is a relatively common condition involving inflammation and sometimes infection of the bursa over the posterior aspect of the elbow. Potential precipitating causes include previous or recurrent trauma, localized infection, or gout.

Presentation

- Painful swelling over posterior aspect of elbow/point of olecranon
- Erythema and heat can be indicative of an infected bursitis:
  - A pointing collection may be seen
- Elbow movement is unusually maintained.

Management

- Conservative:
  - Activity modification
  - Analgesia
  - Aspiration and antibiotics for infection
- Surgical:
  - Rarely indicated apart from refractory infection or chronic bursitis, which can be associated with calcific deposits
  - Washout of bursa +/− excision.

 HINTS AND TIPS

OLECRANON BURSITIS

Elbow movement and function is usually maintained for patients with olecranon bursitis, even when infected. The bursa can be aspirated and sent to microbiology to provide targeted antibiotic therapy. Loss of elbow movement, pyrexia and a universally hot and painful joint is more indicative of a septic arthritis of the elbow. This requires urgent joint washout in theatre.

WRIST AND HAND

Distal Radius Fractures

 OVERVIEW

Distal radius fractures are often seen in elderly osteoporotic postmenopausal women. Assessment must include a full neurovascular assessment of the hand and the integrity of the surrounding skin. Manipulation under regional block or anaesthesia is often the first-line treatment, with displaced unstable fractures requiring surgical intervention depending on the patient's underlying health and functional demands.

Fractures of the distal radius occur following a low-energy fall (FOOSH) in postmenopausal women (where it tends to occur at a younger age than fragility fractures of the hip and spine), or can be associated with higher energy injuries in younger patients. It is the most frequent fracture of the upper limb. The most common type is the Colles type fracture – dorsal angulation and displacement of the distal fragment. A Smith fracture is characterized by a transverse extraarticular distal radial fracture near the radiocarpal joint, with volar angulation and displacement of the distal fragment. It commonly occurs after a fall onto the dorsal aspect of the hand.

Presentation

- Wrist pain and swelling with a restricted range of movement
- 'Dinner-fork' wrist deformity due to shortening (radial) and angulation
- It is essential to assess the neurovascular status of the affected limb:
  - Assess median and ulnar nerve function and radial artery status.

Investigations

- Wrist radiographs (AP and lateral) (Figure 6.5):
  - Look for displacement, angulation, impaction and associated fracture (avulsion, intraarticular, Barton fracture – intraarticular distal radial fracture with dislocation of the radiocarpal joint)

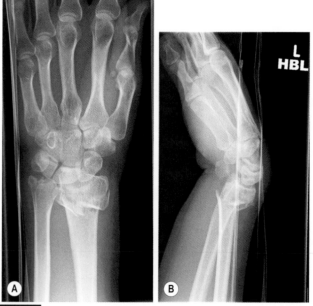

FIGURE 6.5

Comminuted distal radial fracture with dorsal angulation, carpal malalignment, shortening and an associated avulsion fracture of the ulnar styloid. (**A**) AP; (**B**) lateral.

- May still treat even if no fracture seen (clinical fracture)
- Associated ulnar styloid fracture.

Management
- Conservative:
  - Immediate reduction using a regional block (e.g. Bier's) if displaced; remember a check radiograph postreduction (repeated at 1–2 weeks)
  - Immobilization (e.g. Colles cast), total time in cast ~6 weeks
  - Referral to fracture liaison service (see Chapter 5)
  - Physiotherapy
- Surgical:
  - Considered for re-displacement (instability) or for complex fractures (intraarticular, comminuted, open, concomitant carpal injury)
  - Percutaneous K-wire fixation or external fixation for unstable fractures
  - Open reduction and fixation for intraarticular fractures
  - Bone grafting and internal fixation for radial collapse.

Complications
- Postoperative:
  - Infection
  - Flexor tendon rupture, e.g. flexor pollicis longus, following volar plate fixation
  - Removal of metalwork
- Stiffness, pain and deformity:
  - CRPS (see Chapter 5)
  - Malunion often with associated angulation (corrected by osteotomy)
- Neurovascular and soft tissue injury:
  - Median (acute carpal tunnel syndrome) and/or ulnar nerve neurapraxia
  - Radial and/or ulnar artery (rare)
  - Extensor pollicis longus tendon rupture (delayed complication).

 HINTS AND TIPS

DISTAL RADIUS FRACTURES

In elderly lower demand patients there is evidence to suggest that malunion of the distal radius does not lead to a poor patient-reported outcome. Surgery in this patient group for displaced unstable fractures is debated. Volar displaced fractures of the distal radius routinely require surgery with a buttress plate due to instability. Classical sequelae of distal radius malunion and shortening are pain at the distal radial ulnar joint, a reduction in the range of supination, and difficulty with day-to-day activities such as turning a key or opening a tight jar.

 PROCEDURE

MANIPULATION OF A DISTAL RADIUS FRACTURE

CONSENT

- Risk of loss of reduction
- Risk of neurovascular injury
- Pain
- Side effects of anaesthesia/sedation

Continued

PROCEDURE—cont'd

PROCEDURE

Suitable anaesthesia, sedation or regional anaesthesia is required. Grasp the affected hand, encompassing the patient's thumb in one hand and little finger in the other. Apply sustained longitudinal traction (with an assistant applying countertraction to the humerus) until disimpaction of the two fragments is achieved. This is usually appreciated by a distinct 'give' but can otherwise be determined by mobility at the fracture site.

Adjust your grip to allow your thumbs to rest on the distal fragment and use these as a fulcrum to bring the fracture into extension (increasing the deformity). Apply further traction until the dorsal cortex is realigned, and then flex at the fracture site to reduce the distal fragment.

A back slab is applied, with a dorsal back slab for Colles type fractures. Stability of the reduced fracture is principally dictated by the degree of comminution, the patient's age and the reduction achieved. However, key considerations to the back slab are adequate padding to bony prominences, free mobility of the elbow and MCPJs, and avoidance of both excessive wrist flexion and constriction at the base of the thumb.

Scaphoid Fractures

A scaphoid fracture is common after a fall onto the outstretched hand (FOOSH) with a dorsiflexed wrist, accounting for three-quarters of all carpal bone fractures. It is commonly seen in younger patients with a male predominance. It is important not to miss a scaphoid fracture because of the serious potential complications that can ensue if untreated.

Presentation

- All clinical signs have poor diagnostic performance characteristics
- Wrist pain and swelling with sometimes a restricted range of movement
- Tenderness notable on gripping and wrist extension
- Tender and full ASB (anatomical snuff box), the borders of which are:
  - Proximal = radial styloid
  - Posterior/medial = extensor pollicis longus tendon
  - Anterior/lateral = extensor pollicis brevis and abductor pollicis longus tendon
  - Distal = midpoint of the thumb metacarpal
- Multitude of other clinical signs:
  - ASB pain on axial compression of thumb
  - Scaphoid tubercle tenderness
  - ASB pain on ulnar/radial deviation of the wrist
  - ASB pain on thumb–index finger pinch
  - Decreased range of thumb movement
- Assess the neurovascular status of the affected hand.

Investigations

- Scaphoid view radiographs (PA +/– Ziter view, lateral and two obliques):
  - Fracture, most commonly seen at waist (Figure 6.6)

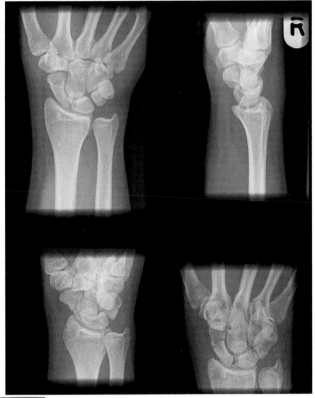

FIGURE 6.6

Fracture through the waist of the right scaphoid (scaphoid radiograph views).

- Less common are proximal pole fractures that are associated with the highest risk of AVN
- Ligament damage along with displacement (widening of space between carpal bones)
- Be sure to rule out a carpal dislocation (see below)
- Repeat radiograph at 2 weeks if fracture not seen and still treat if clinical fracture (see below).
- CT or MRI for the suspected occult fracture or displaced complex fractures.

Management
- Conservative:
  - Immobilization (e.g. Colles or scaphoid cast)
  - A period of up to 12 weeks in a cast is sometimes required

- Suspected scaphoid fractures require splint immobilization or equivalent and review within 2 weeks of injury for further assessment and imaging as above
- Surgical:
  - Considered if there is a proximal pole fracture, instability, displacement, angulation or concomitant carpal dislocation
  - Open reduction and compression screw fixation
  - Bone grafting and internal fixation for delayed or nonunion
  - Percutaneous fixation for undisplaced or minimally displaced fractures is reported to have a shorter time to return to work and sports and a lower nonunion rate, although outcome at 1 year is equivalent.

Complications

- Stiffness and pain
- Neurovascular and soft tissue injury:
  - Trans-scaphoid perilunate dislocation
- AVN (30%):
  - Blood supply occurs from the distal to proximal pole
  - Proximal pole fractures
  - Secondary OA and carpal collapse
- Nonunion:
  - Secondary OA and carpal collapse.

 HINTS AND TIPS

SCAPHOID FRACTURES

The clinical scaphoid fracture continues to be a diagnostic conundrum for orthopaedic surgeons, balancing the risk of unnecessary immobilization in young and active patients with the risk of nonunion if a fracture is missed. The sensitivity and specificity of the clinical tests available is poor, and radiographs have noted limitations. The role of early advanced imaging (e.g. CT or MRI) is advocated by some and others support the use of clinical prediction rules to identify high-risk patients who should undergo such imaging. Litigation can result in cases of missed fractures that result in a non-union.

Carpal Dislocation and Fracture-Dislocation

Carpal dislocations do occur and should not be missed; the most frequent is a lunate or perilunate dislocation or fracture-dislocation. The severity of this is measured by the Mayfield classification.

Presentation

- Frequently occurs following a high-energy fall onto an outstretched hand
- Wrist pain, swelling and deformity can be seen with:
  - Grossly restricted range of movement
- Assessment of neurovascular status is essential:
  - Median nerve injury commonly seen.

Investigations

- AP and lateral wrist radiographs are essential:
  - Scaphoid views if necessary
  - Look for associated fractures of the carpus
- Further imaging as indicated but should not delay immediate reduction.

Management

- Urgent reduction and immobilization:
  - Re-assess neurovascular status (median nerve) post-reduction
- Definitive stabilization, e.g. with K-wire fixation +/– ligament repair +/– carpal bone fixation (e.g. scaphoid screw fixation).

Complications

- Severe ongoing pain and stiffness
- AVN and OA of the lunate
- Neurovascular injury.

Bennett Fracture

Bennett fracture–subluxation/dislocation is a thumb metacarpal base intraarticular fracture with proximal and radial displacement of the major fragment of the metacarpal.

Presentation

- Thumb-base pain and swelling
- Range of movement at the thumb CMCJ is reduced with instability often apparent
- Assess neurovascular status of the affected thumb.

Investigations

- Thumb radiographs (AP, lateral and oblique):
  - Fracture and instability (Figure 6.7)
  - Repeat radiograph at 2 weeks if fracture not seen (scaphoid views to exclude fracture).

Management

- Conservative:
  - Closed reduction with analgesia/ring block
  - Immobilization (e.g. Bennett cast).
- Surgical:
  - Often considered due to instability or malpositioning
  - Open reduction and screw or percutaneous wire fixation.

Complications

- Malunion
- Pain and stiffness:
  - Long-term risk of secondary OA if degree of injury to CMCJ is severe.

Thumb Collateral Ligament Injury (Gamekeeper's Thumb)

Now more commonly known as skier's thumb, this is a rupture of the ulnar collateral ligament (UCL) of the thumb, which originates on the head of the thumb metacarpal and inserts onto the proximal phalanx. If there is a complete rupture of the ligament, some patients may have a Stener lesion. This is interposition of the aponeurosis of the adductor pollicis muscle, with or without an associated fracture, between the insertion and the ruptured free edge of the ligament. Untreated complete ruptures have a poor functional outcome as the UCL is vital to a strong grip.

Presentation

- Common after a fall (abduction force) onto an extended thumb
- Painful, swelling and bruising of the thumb:
  - Ulnar side particularly
- Restricted range of movement
- Tenderness will be noted over the ulnar aspect of the thumb MCPJ
- Attempt to assess both collateral ligaments:
  - Some advocate local anaesthetic injection to aid examination
  - Compare with contralateral side.

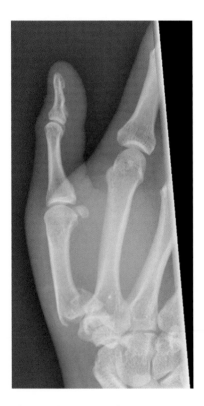

FIGURE 6.7
Bennett fracture–subluxation of the right thumb.

Investigations
- AP and lateral +/− radial stress view radiographs of the thumb:
  - Exclude associated avulsion fracture, e.g. proximal phalanx base.

Management
- Conservative:
  - For partial ruptures with immobilization in a thumb spica/cast
- Surgical:
  - For a complete rupture and/or a fracture.

Metacarpal Fractures

 OVERVIEW

Metacarpal fractures account for 30–50% of all hand fractures and can be differentiated into:

1. Thumb metacarpal head, shaft and base fractures
2. Finger metacarpal head, neck, shaft and base fractures

Clinical assessment needs to assess for clinical deformity and the presence of an open injury. The vast majority of fractures are managed nonoperatively.

Fractures of the fifth metacarpal account for 60% of all injuries. The variety of injury mechanisms leading to fracture range from axial loading due to falls to direct dorsal blows to the hand (boxer's fracture). Associated subsequent deformities of the hand following fracture include shortening, angulation and malrotation, along with soft tissue injury and swelling. The index and middle fingers have less tolerance for deformity than the ring and little fingers.

Presentation
- Metacarpal pain and swelling
- Deformity if displaced fracture:
  - Flattened knuckle or protrusion on dorsal aspect of the hand
  - Scissoring of fingers (rotational deformity)
- Bite marks over fifth knuckle:
  - 'Fight bite', often human and postpunch, prone to aerobic and/or anaerobic infection.

Investigations
- Hand radiograph (AP, lateral and oblique):
  - Fracture and displacement (Figure 6.8).

Management
- Conservative:
  - A vast number of metacarpal fractures are closed injuries, adequately treated by immobilization, with or without closed reduction as necessary
  - Immobilization (e.g. neighbour strapping, plaster as required)
- Surgical:
  - Considered (rare) if there is significant displacement/deformity of the finger

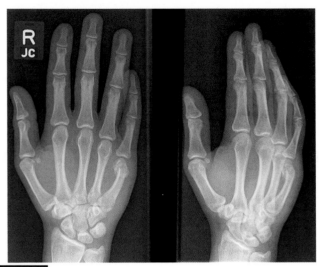

FIGURE 6.8

Fracture of the neck of the fifth metacarpal (boxer's fracture).

- Mandatory exploration and washout if joint is penetrated ('fight bite')
- Percutaneous K-wire fixation
- ORIF is considered for fractures that are unstable, open, multiple, or irreducible closed.

Complications

- Postoperative infection
- Stiffness and pain:
  - OA
- Nonunion
- Malunion:
  - Rotational deformity leading to disability of the hand.

 HINTS AND TIPS

METACARPAL FRACTURES

Hand swelling and stiffness posttrauma (including surgery) can lead to fixed fibrosis and contracture, which can result in severe disability for the patient. Elevation and early movement is key in the management of all forearm, wrist and hand injuries to minimize swelling and prevent stiffness. When splinting the wrist and hand, it is important to do so in a 'position of safety' to avoid contractures. The Edinburgh position involves MCPJ flexion at 90°, with PIPJ and DIPJ in full extension.

Phalangeal Fractures

Fractures and/or dislocations to the phalanges often follow direct trauma, e.g. impact or twisting. Crush fractures of the distal phalanges are not uncommon and may be open but can often be managed expectantly.

Presentation

- Pain, swelling and possibly deformity over the affected finger:
  - Look for any rotational or angulational deformity
- Assess the soft tissues:
  - Flexors and extensors of fingers
- Neurovascular assessment
- Check for open injury.

Investigations

- AP, lateral and oblique views of individual finger:
  - Assess for displacement and instability.

Management

- Conservative:
  - Reduction under block if indicated, check neurovascular status postreduction with check radiographs
  - Splint immobilization, e.g. neighbour strapping
  - Distal phalanx open fractures may require trephining of a subungual haematoma, antibiotics +/− tetanus
- Surgical:
  - For displaced/unstable fractures and those associated with clinical deformity
  - Closed reduction with K-wires is the mainstay
  - Few require open reduction.

 PROCEDURE

METACARPAL AND DIGITAL NERVE BLOCKS

CONSENT

- Pain
- Infection (rare)
- Neurovascular injury (rare)
- Failed reduction or re-displacement

PROCEDURE

In all extremity blocks associated with terminal arteries it is essential to ensure that the anaesthetic being used does not contain adrenaline. A metacarpal block is performed by identifying the soft intermetacarpal space at the midshaft level on either side of the affected finger. Direct the point of the needle from dorsal to palmar aiming to converge towards the midline on the palmar aspect of the bone. Aspirate during needle insertion to ensure extravascular placement. Inject gradually during withdrawal in order to infiltrate the tissues around the metacarpal evenly and circumferentially. A digital block is performed following the same principles on either side of the proximal phalanx of the affected finger.

Mallet Finger

A mallet finger is commonly caused by a direct blow to an actively extended finger, e.g. a cricket ball impacting the end of the finger. This leads to hyperflexion of the distal phalanx and subsequent rupture of the extensor digitorum tendon. An avulsion from the base of the distal phalanx can also occur, and a boutonnière deformity is the presentation when the central slip of the extensor tendon ruptures.

Presentation

- Tenderness and swelling over DIPJ/distal phalanx of affected finger
- Flexible flexion deformity at the DIPJ (passive but NOT active extension possible).

Investigations

- AP, lateral +/– oblique views of the affected finger:
  - Exclude associated fracture.

Management

- Conservative:
  - Splint immobilization (mallet splint) of the DIPJ in hyperextension
- Surgical:
  - Fixation (extension blocking wire) is indicated if there is significantly displaced fracture +/– subluxation of the joint
  - Fusion may be required if there is a severe deformity postsplintage.

HINTS AND TIPS

MALLET FINGER

A boutonnière deformity occurs when the extensor tendon central slip ruptures. A mallet thumb is caused by rupture of the EPL tendon, due to a variety of causes, e.g. direct trauma, post distal radius fracture and RA. A free tendon transfer (e.g. extensor indicis) can be required in chronic cases.

Carpal Tunnel Syndrome

Carpal tunnel syndrome is the most common compressive neuropathy. It is caused by compression and subsequent ischaemia of the median nerve as it enters the hand under the flexor retinaculum (transverse carpal ligament) of the carpal tunnel (Figure 6.9). Middle-aged women (8:1) are most commonly affected. Risk factors include:

- Fluid retention: pregnancy and combined oral contraceptive pill
- Musculoskeletal: RA or OA
- Endocrine: diabetes mellitus, obesity, hypothyroidism, myxoedema, acromegaly and congestive cardiac failure
- Trauma: distal radius or carpal bone fracture/dislocation, e.g. lunate
- Occupation (debated).

Presentation

- Paraesthesia of the median distribution (thumb, index, middle and the radial half of the ring fingers):
  - More marked at night

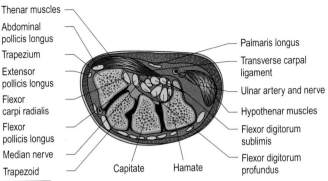

Thenar muscles
Abdominal pollicis longus
Trapezium
Extensor pollicis longus
Flexor carpi radialis
Flexor pollicis longus
Median nerve
Trapezoid

Palmaris longus
Transverse carpal ligament
Ulnar artery and nerve
Hypothenar muscles
Flexor digitorum sublimis
Flexor digitorum profundus

Capitate   Hamate

FIGURE 6.9

Cross-sectional anatomy of the carpal tunnel.

- Often relieved by shaking the hand ('flick sign')
- Can radiate up the forearm
- Perception of pain in CTS is a complex phenomenon and is secondary to paraethesia
- Lateral aspect of palm spared as superficial palmar branch is given off proximal to flexor retinaculum.
- Thenar muscle wasting (advanced cases):
  - Abductor pollicis brevis weakness.
- Phalen test (hyperflexed wrist for 2 minutes will reproduce symptoms).
- Tinel test (tapping in region of nerve on anterior wrist crease) is less sensitive.

Investigations

Nerve conduction studies advocated by some and usually reveal some median nerve deficit.

Management

- Conservative:
  - Splint immobilization at night (extension wrist splints)
  - Corticosteroid injection (diagnostic)
- Surgical:
  - Carpal tunnel decompression by flexor retinaculum division.

Complications

- Postoperative:
  - Pillar pain
  - Scar sensitivity
  - Infection
  - Neurovascular injury (rare).

HINTS AND TIPS

CARPAL TUNNEL SYNDROME

Paraesthesia of the hand can often be mistaken as pain, but pain is not a classical symptom of carpal tunnel syndrome. The diagnosis is often made using a combination of clinical symptoms and signs, and nerve conduction studies. Nerve conduction studies can rule out other neuropathies both proximally and distally, particularly if the clinical picture is nonspecific.

 PROCEDURE

CARPAL TUNNEL INJECTION

CONSENT

- Risk of infection (rare)
- Risk of neurovascular injury (rare)
- Risk of no benefit

PROCEDURE

Palpate the distal pole of the scaphoid and the pisiform and place the needle at the midpoint and pass perpendicularly from palmar to dorsal. Use caution to feel the needle passing through the palmar fascia and then the resistance of the transverse carpal ligament. Stop advancing as soon as this resistance is lost and inject into the carpal tunnel superficial to the median nerve. If a sharp pain or symptoms in the median nerve distribution is precipitated, withdraw the needle and do not inject.

 PROCEDURE

CARPAL TUNNEL DECOMPRESSION

CONSENT

- Risk of infection
- Risk of reduced grip strength
- Risk of pillar pain (pain leaning on a dorsiflexed wrist)
- Risk of failure to alleviate symptoms
- Risk of neurovascular damage (including palmar cutaneous sensory branch)

PROCEDURE

The procedure can be performed under LA or GA, with a tourniquet applied to the upper arm but not inflated if under LA. A longitudinal incision is made in a line between the middle and the ring finger, stretching distally from the wrist crease. It should proceed no further than an imaginary line (Kaplan's line) running transversely from the thumb metacarpophalangeal joint. This prevents incursion into the dangerous territory beyond where the radial artery communicates with the arterial palmar arches. Dissection continues in a sharp manner through the palmar subcutaneous fat layer. Exposure is aided by inserting a self-retaining retractor. Dissection then reveals the transverse carpal ligament.

The ligament is carefully incised in its distal portion initially until the incision is large enough to pass a McDonald dissector underneath the ligament to protect the median nerve. The ligament is incised directly onto the McDonald dissector working in a proximal and then distal direction. Care should be taken to avoid the palmar cutaneous sensory branch of the median nerve (proximally) and the vascular arches distally. Ensure complete release before closing with simple interrupted nylon sutures.

Dupuytren's Contracture

 OVERVIEW

Dupuytren's contracture, first described in 1831 by a Parisian surgeon, is a progressive, painless fibrotic thickening of the palmar and digital fascia (aponeurosis), leading to nodular hypertrophy and contracture of the fascia. There is a strong genetic component. Deformity but not pain is the common presentation. Management is dependent on the disability and severity of the disease.

The clinical picture of Dupuytren's is a hand contracture that commences often at the base of the ring and little finger, leading to skin puckering and tethering, with fixed flexion deformity of the affected fingers. It is more common in men (10:1) and between the ages of 40 and 60 years. Risk factors include:

- Family history (autosomal dominant pattern)
- Alcoholism and liver disease
- Smoking
- Epilepsy/antiepileptic drugs, e.g. phenytoin therapy
- Endocrine, e.g. diabetes mellitus, hypothyroidism
- AIDS/HIV
- Trauma/postsurgery.

Presentation
- Bilateral and symmetrical
- Pain uncommon
- Puckered, nodular thickening of the palm
- Contracture of the MCPJ and PIPJ of the ring and little fingers
- Hueston tabletop test is positive, i.e. cannot place hand flat and open on table
- Associated presentations:
  - Garrod knuckle pads: thickened skin over the dorsum of the PIPJ
  - Ledderhose disease: plantar fascia thickening
  - Peyronie disease: penile fibromatosis resulting in curvature.

Management
- Conservative:
  - None effective
  - Collagenase therapy (benefits debated)
- Surgical:
  - Considered if patient is disabled with deformity
  - Fasciotomy, fasciectomy or dermofasciectomy +/– skin grafting
  - Postoperative splinting and physiotherapy
  - Digital amputation if severe.

Complications
- Recurrence is common
- Postoperative:
  - Infection
  - Neurovascular injury
  - Swelling due to oedema and haematoma

- Stiffness and pain:
  - CRPS
  - Loss of function.

De Quervain's Tenosynovitis

De Quervain's tenosynovitis, first described in 1895 by Swiss surgeon Fritz de Quervain, is an inflammation and stenosis of the tendon sheaths of abductor pollicis longus and extensor pollicis brevis (first extensor compartment). Inflammation and pain commonly occur secondary to a repetitive movement. It is also associated with inflammatory arthritis and is commonly seen in middle-aged women (30–50 years). Potential risk factors include pregnancy, repetitive microtrauma and inflammatory arthropathies.

Presentation

- Wrist and thumb pain on use, but often with full range of movement
- Pain at the site of inflammation, as the tendons pass between the radial styloid and the overlying extensor retinaculum:
  - Crepitus sometimes felt
- Finkelstein test reproduces the pain:
  - Flexion of the thumb across the palm
  - Encompass with fist
  - Then ulnar deviation of the wrist.

Investigations

Radiograph of thumb can be indicated to rule out bony pathology, e.g. CMCJ OA.

Management

- Conservative:
  - Activity modification and splints
  - Analgesia, e.g. NSAIDs
  - Corticosteroid injection
- Surgical:
  - Division and release of the tendon sheath of the first dorsal compartment.

Complications

- Postoperative:
  - Superficial radial nerve neurapraxia/injury
- Radiocarpal instability
- Recurrence.

Trigger Finger

Triggering can affect the fingers or thumb and commonly affects women between 40 and 60 years of age. It is caused by tendon sheath inflammation and subsequent fibrotic thickening, which results in a tendon–sheath size mismatch. This stenosis leads to restricted movement and eventual entrapment of the flexor tendon within the retinacular pulley. This is commonly found at the first annular (A1) pulley of the ring or middle fingers. Risk factors include diabetes, RA, amyloidosis and gout.

Presentation

- History of the finger becoming locked in a flexed position:
  - Digit locked in flexion on attempt at passive extension
  - Unlocked forcibly by patient
- Tender nodule flexor aspect of the affected finger/thumb.

Management

- Conservative:
  - Physiotherapy
  - Steroid injection
- Surgical:
  - Indicated for refractory cases
  - Release +/− debride pulley.

PELVIS, HIP AND KNEE

Pelvic and Acetabular Fractures

 OVERVIEW

Fractures to the pelvic ring or acetabulum commonly occur following high energy injuries e.g. RTAs, or when elderly people sustain a simple low energy fall (pubic rami fractures). All fractures, but particularly complex unstable fractures, are associated with considerable blood loss. Displacement of the pelvis can lead to urogenital injury.

Presentation

- Pain and bruising in the pelvic region
- Flank, perianal and urogenital swelling, bruising and bleeding
- Per rectum examination may reveal a high-riding prostate
- It is essential to assess the distal neurology:
  - In particular, assess the sciatic and inferior/superior gluteal nerves.

Investigations

- Pelvic radiograph (AP, inlet, outlet and oblique views):
  - Young–Burgess classification (lateral compression, AP compression, vertical shear, combined)
  - Tile classification
- CT of the pelvis:
  - Often definitive
  - Urogenital assessment possible.

Management

- ATLS assessment and resuscitation
- Pelvic stabilization using a pelvic binder or rarely now an external fixator (prevents clot disruption and thus helps to control haemorrhage):
  - Radiological embolization may be required to control haemorrhage
- Surgical:
  - Definitive fixation individualized to patient and fracture
  - Often indicated for unstable pelvic fractures and for displaced acetabular fractures.

Complications

- Persistent pain, stiffness and instability
- Malunion and OA (acetabular fractures):
  - Conversion to total hip replacement potentially required
- Urogenital and rectal injury with dysfunction
- Neurovascular injury:
  - Sciatic nerve and nerve roots.

Hip Dislocation

Hip dislocation is commonly characterized by a posterior displacement of the femoral head following a blow to the thigh with the hip in flexion and adduction, e.g. a direct blow to the knee on a dashboard.

Presentation

- Hip pain and swelling with a restricted range of movement.
- Gross deformity often apparent:
  - Loss of normal skin crease
  - Posterior: hip is flexed, adducted, shortened and internally rotated
  - Anterior: hip is flexed, abducted and externally rotated
- It is essential to assess the neurovascular status of the affected limb before and after reduction:
  - In particular, assess the sciatic nerve.

Investigations

- Hip, femur and knee radiographs (AP and lateral):
  - Position of dislocation (Thompson–Epstein classification)
  - Coexisting injury, e.g. acetabular fracture, femoral head fracture (Pipkin classification), femoral shaft fracture, and PCL injury of the knee
- CT pelvis following reduction:
  - Now routine practice to assess for reduction of the hip joint and for associated bony injuries

Management

- Conservative (no fracture):
  - Immediate reduction under GA; remember a check radiograph + CT scan postreduction
  - Immobilization (rest)
  - Physiotherapy
- Surgical:
  - Considered for fracture-dislocations, e.g. displaced fracture of acetabulum or a femoral head/neck fracture.

Complications

- Recurrence
- Avascular necrosis of femoral head:
  - Secondary OA
- Neurovascular injury:
  - Sciatic nerve.

Proximal Femoral Fractures

 OVERVIEW

Fractures of the femoral neck are often caused by a direct blow to the hip and occur most commonly following a minor trauma (e.g. fall) in the elderly (chiefly postmenopausal osteoporotic women). Rarely, they occur following severe trauma (e.g. RTA) in the young. Surgical management with fixation or replacement is the mainstay of treatment. Mortality is quoted as approximately 30% within 12 months of the fracture.

Fractures of the femoral neck are a common geriatric osteoporotic fracture. The blood supply to the femoral head makes it vulnerable to developing avascular necrosis. The primary vasculatures (retinacular branches of medial circumflex femoral artery and medullary vessels) are damaged severely if there is a displaced intracapsular fracture of the neck, leading to avascular necrosis (AVN) and collapse of the femoral head. Extracapsular hip fractures do not disturb the blood supply to the femoral head and commonly occur between the greater and the lesser trochanters, i.e. intertrochanteric fractures. Less common are subtrochanteric fractures.

Presentation

- History of trauma
- Hip pain with little or no weight bearing or movement possible
- Displaced fractures cause external rotation and shortening of the leg.

Investigations

- Hip and pelvic radiographs (AP and lateral) (Figure 6.10):
  - Shenton's line (really a parabolic curve) runs along the upper border of the obturator foramen and the inferior border of the femoral neck; an

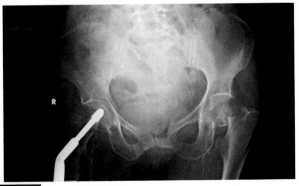

FIGURE 6.10

An intracapsular fracture of the left neck of the femur. There is a dynamic hip screw (DHS) in place for an old extracapsular fracture on the right side.

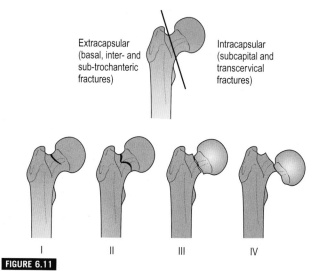

FIGURE 6.11

Garden classification: I, impacted incomplete fracture; II, nondisplaced complete fracture; III, partially displaced complete fracture; IV, fully displaced complete fracture. The closer the fracture is to the head, the more likely the retinacular vessels will be disrupted leading to AVN. Displaced fractures are associated with an increased risk of complications and avascular necrosis.

alteration in this line will identify any possible fracture and displacement of the hip
- Garden classification of hip fractures is shown in Figure 6.11.

Management
- ATLS assessment and resuscitation; assess for precipitating events (e.g. MI, stroke, infection)
- If surgery contraindicated (very rare due to higher mortality), analgesia, rest and chest physiotherapy
- Surgery (Figure 6.12):
  - Intracapsular: hemi-arthroplasty (Figure 6.13), total hip replacement or fixation (young patients)
  - Extracapsular intertrochanteric: dynamic hip screw
  - Extracapsular subtrochanteric: intramedullary nail.

Complications
- Perioperative (see Chapter 4):
  - DVT/PE, pneumonia, renal failure, MI and stroke
- Post-hemi-arthroplasty complications (see Hip and Knee Arthroplasty section in this chapter)
- Death (10% at 1 month, 20% at 3 months, 30% at 1 year)

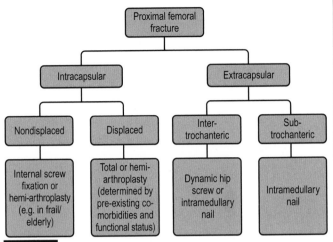

FIGURE 6.12
Surgical options for proximal femoral fractures. Younger patients with a displaced intracapsular fracture can be suitable for early reduction and internal fixation with cannulated screws or equivalent. *(Adapted from Figure 43.1 in Datta PK, Bulstrode CJK, Wallace WFM. MRCS Part A: 500 SBAs and EMQs. 1st edition. JP Medical Publishers; 2012.)*

- Nonunion and malunion leading to secondary OA
- Femoral head avascular necrosis:
  - Increased risk with displaced intracapsular fractures in the young.

 HINTS AND TIPS

PROXIMAL FEMORAL FRACTURES

The prosthesis for hemi-arthroplasty can be either unipolar or bipolar and either cemented or uncemented. During the consent process, it is important to counsel patients and their families about the general mortality after neck of femur fractures, as well as the general medical complications that can occur. Specific complications include infection, thromboembolism, neurovascular injury, dislocation and component failure/removal of metalwork.

Femoral Shaft Fractures

Fractures of the femoral shaft occur following low-energy falls in elderly patients or following high-energy injuries, e.g. RTAs, in younger patients. They are associated with a notable blood loss.

Presentation

- Pain, deformity and bruising in the thigh region
- Assess the soft tissues of the affected leg

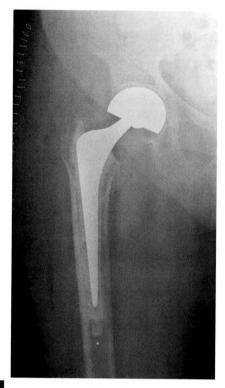

A cemented right bipolar hemi-arthroplasty.

- Knee ligament assessment if possible (may be done intraoperatively)
- Other injuries to the skeleton
- Neurovascular assessment:
  - Sciatic nerve and peripheral circulation.

Investigations
- Femoral AP and lateral radiographs:
  - Ensure hip and knee are visualized.

Management
- Initial resuscitation and temporary fracture splinting, e.g. Thomas splint + traction
- Surgery (intramedullary nail commonly):
  - Antegrade (most common, piriformis or trochanteric entry) and retrograde possible

- ORIF or minimally invasive plating used for some distal femoral or periprosthetic fractures
- Important to assess knee ligament stability and rotation intraoperatively.

Complications

- Postoperative:
  - Infection
  - HO
  - Neurovascular injury
  - Malalignment or malrotation
- Delayed union, malunion and nonunion
- Fat embolism
- Pain and stiffness.

Knee Ligament Injuries

 OVERVIEW

Knee ligament injuries can occur following a twist or a direct blow to the medial or lateral aspect of the knee. A feeling of instability and a rapidly developing effusion is often associated with a cruciate ligament injury as they are highly vascular (haemarthrosis). The most important aspect of classifying a ligament injury is whether there is tenderness around the ligament insertions (collaterals), if there is an increased laxity of the ligament and whether there is a firm endpoint to testing. Diagnosis is routinely a combination of clinical assessment, radiographs of the knee to exclude a bony injury, and MRI. Conservative management with physiotherapy may suffice for some, with reconstruction reserved for persistent instability and high-level athletes.

For the assessment and management of specific knee ligament injuries see Table 6.3.

 HINTS AND TIPS

KNEE LIGAMENT INJURIES

Examining a patient with a suspected knee ligament injury can often be difficult in the immediate acute phase following injury. There is a benefit to re-examining the patient after a period of rest, in order to allow any effusion to subside. When laxity is suspected it is important to compare this with the contralateral knee. Laxity of a collateral ligament in full knee extension is indicative of an associated cruciate ligament injury. Isolated collateral ligament laxity is best assessed with the knee in 10–20° of flexion. Knee ligament injuries are often associated with other ligament injuries to the knee, i.e. multiligament, and concomitant meniscal injuries.

Meniscal Injuries

 OVERVIEW

Damage to these fibrocartilaginous load-bearing structures can be acute (normal menisci, damage due to twisting, common following sports injury) or chronic (abnormal menisci, damage after little trauma, common in the elderly). Diagnosis is made clinically in conjunction with MRI.

TABLE 6.3

THE AETIOLOGY, PRESENTATION AND MANAGEMENT OF KNEE LIGAMENT INJURIES

Complications of conservative treatment are recurrent instability and secondary OA. Complications of surgery include pain and stiffness, patella injury, infection, residual symptoms, recurrent instability and secondary OA.

Aetiology	Presentation and Investigations	Management
ACL		
More common in males Incidence 1 in 3000/year Common sports injury Valgus twisting, hyperextension, foot rigid to ground, knee flexed Associated ligament (MCL) and menisci (lateral more common than medial) injury	History of trauma Effusion and pain Decreased ROM Positive anterior draw test/Lachmann Positive pivot shift test MRI +/− arthroscopy	Rest and analgesia Physiotherapy Ligament reconstruction Repair meniscal tear
PCL		
Uncommon (5–20% of all knee ligament injuries) Common following RTAs (knee flexed, tibia forced posteriorly) Other ligament injury very common	Missed diagnosis acutely History of trauma Inability to weight bear, knee gives way Positive posterior draw test MRI +/− arthroscopy	Rest and analgesia Physiotherapy Ligament reconstruction (rare)
MCL		
Most common Associated ACL or medial meniscal injury Lateral blow is common (valgus stress)	History of trauma Effusion uncommon Tenderness Valgus testing positive (grade 1–3) MRI to confirm	Rest and analgesia Physiotherapy Immobilization if needed Surgery if unstable or chronic
LCL		
Uncommon Medial blow is common (varus stress) Associated with ACL and PCL injury Associated with biceps femoris tendon, fascia lata and common peroneal nerve injury	Instability less common LCL not easily found Varus testing positive (grade 1–3) MRI to confirm	Rest and analgesia Physiotherapy Immobilization if needed Surgery rarely needed

Meniscal injuries can occur with high-level activities such as sports, but may also occur in the degenerative knee. Men are more frequently affected. The medial meniscus is more commonly affected than the lateral due to its decreased mobility in relation to the capsule. However, a lateral meniscal injury will more likely lead to degenerative changes due to the convex shape of the lateral tibial plateau. Six types of meniscal tear are:

- Radial
- Bucket-handle
- Flap

- Horizontal cleavage (common in degenerated menisci)
- Vertical
- Degenerative.

The position of the tear is of clinical relevance in terms of ability to heal due to varying vascular supply, i.e. the more peripheral the tear the greater the chance of repair due to an increased vascular supply.

Presentation

- Joint line pain and tenderness
- A locked knee:
  - Unable to fully extend passively or actively
- Swelling (effusion)
- McMurray or Apley test: positive in up to 70%
- Positive squat test
- Associated ligament injury may be present.

Investigations

MRI and arthroscopy can be used to confirm the diagnosis.

Management

- Conservative:
  - Rest, analgesia and physiotherapy
- Surgery:
  - Indicated for the symptomatic/locked knee
  - Arthroscopy involves either repair or partial meniscectomy.

Complications

- Postoperative:
  - Infection (<1%)
  - Residual/recurrent symptoms
- OA, particularly in large meniscectomies.

 HINTS AND TIPS

MENISCAL INJURIES

Meniscal injuries often present with a slow developing effusion and potentially a locked knee, with joint line tenderness on the side of the injury. In the acute setting, the patient may have been able to continue the activity they were doing, e.g. football, with the symptoms developing hours later.

Patella Fractures

Patella fractures are more common in males and occur most commonly between 20 and 50 years of age. Brisk contraction of the quadriceps against resistance can lead to an avulsion or transverse fracture. Direct trauma can also occur secondary to a fall or higher energy injury, e.g. from the dashboard in an RTA. Patella sleeve fractures can occur in children.

Presentation

- Pain, swelling and bruising over anterior aspect of the knee:
  - Palpable defect in patella

- Reduced range of movement:
  - Essential to assess ability to straight leg raise
- Assess skin for open injuries
- Assess for proximal injury to femur or hip in high-energy injuries
- Neurovascular assessment.

Investigations

- AP and lateral views of knee:
  - Assess for articular incongruity on lateral view.

Management

- Conservative:
  - Undisplaced fractures that do not affect the extensor mechanism (patient can straight leg raise)
  - Immobilization of the knee in extension
  - Combination of cylinder cast and knee bracing
- Surgical:
  - Displaced fractures and disruption of extensor mechanism
  - ORIF with tension band wiring, screw and/or wire fixation are potential options
  - Patellectomy (partial) very rarely required for unreconstructable fractures.

Complications

- Postoperative:
  - Infection
  - Metalwork removal
- Pain and stiffness:
  - Anterior knee pain most common
- Nonunion
- AVN (rare):
  - Proximal fragment
- OA of the patellofemoral compartment.

 HINTS AND TIPS

PATELLA FRACTURES

A normal variant on an AP knee radiograph is a congenital bi- or tripartite patella. This can be mistaken for a fracture but often occurs bilaterally.

Extensor Mechanism Injury

Extensor mechanism injuries (excluding a patella fracture) are due to rupture of the patellar tendon (ligamentum patellae) or quadriceps muscle/tendon. Fracture of the patella may present similarly. It is common after a fall onto a flexed knee.

Presentation

- Knee pain, swelling, tenderness and a gap at the point of rupture
- Inability to straight leg raise is common if complete disruption.

Investigations
- Knee radiograph (AP and lateral):
  - Patella is high (patella alta = patella tendon rupture) or low (patella baja = quadriceps tear).

Management
- Conservative:
  - Intact extensor mechanism (patient can straight leg raise)
  - Immobilization of knee in extension
- Surgical:
  - Disrupted extensor mechanism (patient unable to straight leg raise)
  - Repair for tendon rupture +/− avulsion (e.g. from the tibial tubercle).

Dislocation of the Patella

Dislocation of the patella, and subsequent rupture of the medial quadriceps retinaculum and medial patellofemoral ligament, is seen when athletes 'side-step'. It is also seen commonly in teenage girls in whom recurrent dislocations may occur, either spontaneously or with minimal trauma. There are several anatomical variants that predispose to recurrent dislocations (seen after 15–20% of patellar dislocations): ligament laxity, flattening of the lateral epicondyle (trochlear dysplasia), genu valgum, femoral anteversion, external tibial torsion and a small high-riding patella.

Presentation
- Pain, swelling and reduced range of movement:
  - Obvious deformity to knee with patella often found laterally displaced
- Spontaneous reduction at scene is common:
  - Patient presents with swollen painful knee but patella is enlocated
- Positive patella apprehension once acute episode is settled.

Investigations
- Knee AP and lateral radiograph:
  - Exclude an osteochondral fracture
- MRI:
  - Low threshold in younger patients.

Management
- Reduction in the emergency department with lateral displacement of the patella reduced by medial pressure and knee extension under analgesia/sedation:
  - Check radiograph postreduction
- Immobilization and rest with physiotherapy to strengthen the quadriceps
- Surgery in patients with large osteochondral defects or in refractory/recurrent cases.

HINTS AND TIPS

DISLOCATION OF THE PATELLA

It is common for patients and doctors to use the term knee dislocation for a patella dislocation. It is important to be precise and differentiate between a patella dislocation and a dislocation of the knee. A knee dislocation is a severe high-energy injury that results in multiligamentous disruption of the knee and frequently an acute neurovascular compromise to the lower limb. In the case of recurrent patella instability, the lateral radiograph can be used to assess patella height e.g. Insall-Salvati ratio, whilst full length views of the leg can be used to assess for an increased Q-angle (angle between lines from ASIS to centre of patella and centre of patella to tibial tuberosity).

Tibial Plateau Fractures

This injury is often due to a direct compression, i.e. impaction of femoral condyle into the tibial plateau. Damage to either (lateral more common than medial) or both of the tibial condyles is often caused by compression from the opposite femoral condyle.

Presentation
- Knee pain, swelling (haemarthrosis) and deformity (valgus or varus)
- Associated ligament injury may be apparent on testing.

Investigations
- Knee AP and lateral radiographs will show the extent of the fracture:
  - Schatzker classification (types 1–6)
- CT often required for preoperative planning.

Management
- Dependent on the degree of displacement and the extent of fracture(s)
- Conservative:
  - For undisplaced fractures or when surgery is contraindicated
  - Knee bracing +/– casting
- Surgical:
  - ORIF +/– grafting.

Complications
- Postoperative:
  - Acute compartment syndrome (ACS)
  - Neurovascular injury
  - Infection
  - Loss of reduction
- Pain and stiffness
- OA:
  - Small number progress to knee arthroplasty.

Tibial Shaft Fractures

This fracture is often due to a direct or indirect injury. Open fractures do occur along with a concomitant fibula fracture.

Presentation
- Leg pain, swelling and deformity
- Assess for compartment syndrome (see Chapter 4)
- Neurovascular assessment
- Skin assessment.

Investigations
- Leg AP and lateral radiographs:
  - Must include knee and ankle.

Management
- Surgery for vast majority of cases unless completely undisplaced (rare) or patient not fit for surgery:
  - Tibial nail commonly used
  - External fixator
  - Plate fixation predominantly reserved for plateau and pilon fractures.

Complications
- Infection
- Soft tissue and neurovascular injury
- ACS
- Delayed union and nonunion:
  - Increased risk with an open fracture.

Hip and Knee Arthroplasty

 OVERVIEW

Arthroplasty, meaning 'joint changes shape', is the removal or replacement of part, or all, of a particular joint in the body, such as the hip or knee. There are many different types of arthroplasty (excision, unicompartmental, resurfacing, hemi, total), with total hip (Figure 6.14) and knee replacement (Figure 6.15) surgery most common.

The most common indication for hip or knee joint replacement surgery is OA (see Chapter 5). OA can be classified as either primary, i.e. idiopathic, or secondary, e.g. posttraumatic. Other common indications are:

- Fracture:
  - Intracapsular fractures of the proximal femur in high-demand patients
- RA
- Late complication of paediatric hip disorders, e.g. DDH, Perthes disease, SUFE
- Avascular necrosis (see Chapter 4).

The symptoms and signs that indicate joint replacement surgery is required are rest pain, night pain and disability that are refractory to analgesia and other conservative measures, such as lifestyle modification (e.g. weight loss), physiotherapy and walking aids. It is important that these findings correlate with radiographs. The classic features of OA are:

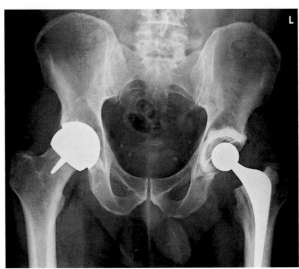

FIGURE 6.14
AP pelvis X-ray demonstrating a cemented left total hip replacement with a right resurfacing hip replacement.

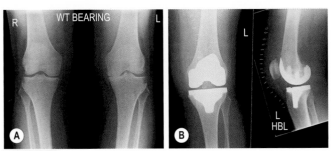

FIGURE 6.15
(**A**) AP standing X-ray of both knees demonstrating medial compartment arthritis with varus deformity of the left knee. (**B**) AP and lateral X-rays of the left knee following a cemented knee replacement.

- Joint space narrowing
- Subchondral sclerosis and cysts
- Osteophyte formation.

Hip Arthroplasty

Hip arthritis is seen in up to a quarter of people over the age of 65 years. Total hip replacement is one of the most successful operations in orthopaedics and the whole of surgery, with satisfaction rates at 90–95% and good longevity reported. A range of bearing surfaces are available that can be cemented or uncemented:

- Metal on polyethylene (well-established)
- Ceramic on polyethylene
- Ceramic on ceramic
- Metal and metal (concerns over elevated metal ion levels, pseudo tumours, early failure).

The classical presentation of hip arthritis is:

- Groin pain that radiates down the anterior thigh to the knee
- Pain is activity related with an associated decline in mobility
- Irritable stiff hip on examination (see Chapter 2):
  - Loss of internal rotation
  - Leg length discrepancy
  - Fixed flexion deformity
  - Antalgic or Trendelenburg gait.

Lateral hip pain can occur, but may be more indicative of lateral trochanteric pain. Spine pathology can lead to hip and leg pain and it is important to differentiate what is the main contributing factor to the patient's symptoms, as these can often coexist. A hip injection walking test can be a useful diagnostic tool in this situation, where LA +/– steroid are injected into the joint under radiological guidance.

APPROACHES
- Lateral/Hardinge:
  - Intramuscular plane splitting gluteus medius (and detaching minimus) and vastus lateralis
  - Structures at potential risk: superior gluteal nerve when splitting proximally; femoral nerve secondary to retractors
- Posterior:
  - Intramuscular plane splitting gluteus maximus and detaching of the piriformis and short external rotators
  - Structures at potential risk: sciatic nerve due to nature of approach; superior gluteal artery and nerve when splitting proximally; and femoral nerve secondary to retractors.

COMPLICATIONS
- Neurovascular injury (<1%):
  - Sciatic nerve (posterior approach)
  - Superior gluteal nerve (lateral approach)
  - Femoral vessels
- Intraoperative fracture (<1%)
- Blood loss:
  - Risk of transfusion (low)
- Persistent pain and/or stiffness (<5%)
- Leg length discrepancy >1 cm (2–5%)

- Infection (<1–2%):
  - Common organisms are coagulase-negative staphylococci (*Staphylococcus epidermidis*) and coagulase-positive staphylococci (*Staphylococcus aureus*)
  - Risks factors are similar to native joint infection (see below) but it is important to consider a history of early wound complications
  - Early prosthetic loosening can occur, predicating that revision surgery includes removal of implants
  - Treatment can range from antibiotics to excision arthroplasty (e.g. Girdlestone procedure for an infected hip prosthesis)
  - A single (debridement, removal of implants, microbiology samples sent, re-implantation of prosthesis) or two-stage (re-implantation of prosthesis occurs at delayed second operation) revision can be performed
  - Prevention is best practice via dedicated elective orthopaedic wards, aseptic and precise surgical techniques, positive-pressure air flow operating theatres and perioperative antibiotics
- Aseptic loosening and wear (2–5%)
- Dislocation of the hip (1–2%)
- Periprosthetic fracture (Figure 6.16)
- Heterotopic ossification (HO)
- General medical complications (see Chapter 4):
  - Infection, e.g. LRTI or UTI
  - MI
  - DVT (2–4%) or PE (<1%) (DVT prophylaxis is essential)
- Death (<1%).

 PROCEDURE

RELOCATION OF DISLOCATED PROSTHETIC HIP

CONSENT

- Risk of periprosthetic fracture
- Risk of neurovascular injury
- Risk of failure and requirement for an open reduction
- Risk of re-dislocation

PROCEDURE

Following the administration of sedation the patient is placed in a supine position. The hip will likely dislocate in the direction of the approach, e.g. posterior approach = posterior dislocation. For the more common posterior dislocation, the hip and knee should be flexed to 90° and longitudinal traction applied to the femur, whilst an assistant provides countertraction by applying pressure to the anterior superior iliac spines with the palms of both hands. A combination of internal and external rotation allows disengagement of the prosthetic head from behind the pelvis and subsequent reduction. For the less common anterior dislocation, longitudinal traction, 20° of abduction and gentle internal rotation are usually successful. Use of a GA with reduction under image intensifier guidance may be required when reduction does not occur easily. The stability of the hip should be assessed (move in standard arc and note when potentially unstable) prior to placing the leg into a temporary anti-dislocation brace e.g. knee extension splint. Subsequent supervised mobilization with physiotherapy should include repeat education regarding the positions of risk.

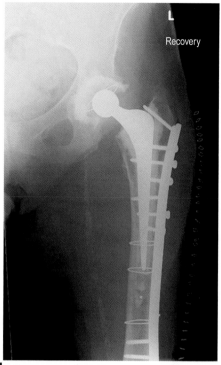

FIGURE 6.16

A periprosthetic fracture around the stem of a cemented total hip replacement that has been managed with open reduction and internal fixation using a plate and cerclage wires.

Knee Arthroplasty

Satisfaction rates following knee replacement (Figure 6.15) are less than hip replacement surgery, at 80–85%, but with good longevity reported. The primary aims of knee replacement surgery include pain relief with sound mechanical re-alignment and balancing of the knee and normal patellofemoral tracking.

In younger patients with isolated medial or lateral compartment OA and a good range of movement, a high tibial osteotomy may avoid or delay the need for a knee replacement. This aims to re-align the joint mechanics so the load is predominantly passing through the unaffected side of the knee. Alternatively, in younger patients with isolated medial compartment arthritis in a stable knee and intact cruciate and collateral ligaments (ACL essential), and minimal varus or FFD (<10–15°) a unicompartmental knee replacement is an option.

Patients with arthritis of the knee often present with:

- Well-localized knee pain
- Reduced range of movement with possible FFD
- Associated coronal deformities:
  - Varus malalignment secondary to medial compartment OA
- Patellofemoral crepitus
- Radiographs of the knee:
  - Should assess all three compartments (medial, lateral, patellofemoral) as well as the overall alignment.

Complications
- Neurovascular injury
- Intraoperative fracture
- Persistent pain and/or stiffness (10–15%):
  - Commoner with knee than hip arthroplasty
- Infection (<1–2%)
  - Management is similar to hip arthroplasty, however, excision arthroplasty is not a viable option and amputation is a possibility in refractory cases
- Aseptic loosening and wear
- Periprosthetic fracture
- General medical complications:
  - Infection, e.g. LRTI or UTI
  - MI/DVT/PE
- Death (<1%).

HINTS AND TIPS

HIP AND KNEE ARTHROPLASTY

During the process of obtaining consent from a patient about to undergo minor or major surgery, it is standard to discuss all severe or major complications, e.g. death, and any other complications with a rate >1%. It is important to make it clear to the patient that a hip injection walking test is a diagnostic and not curative procedure; the patient should keep a diary to document the relief they get from the injection. Although steroid injections in the knee can be effective in controlling symptoms (particularly in those with an effusion), effectiveness often diminishes with time.

ANKLE AND FOOT

Ankle Ligament Sprain

Lateral sprains are most common and are characterized by damage to the anterior talofibular and calcaneofibular ligaments due to talus inversion during trauma. Lateral sprains are more common. Patients can present after a simple twist (often inversion) of the ankle and foot while walking or running.

Presentation
- Ankle pain, swelling and tenderness:
  - Symptoms may be similar to a fracture
- Lateral tenderness and swelling is more common.

Investigations

- AP and lateral radiographs of the ankle as indicated:
  - See Chapter 3 for Ottawa Ankle Rules.

Management

- Conservative:
  - Rest, ice, compression and elevation (RICE), analgesia and immobilization as required
- Surgery:
  - For recurrent instability (rare)
  - Reconstruction +/– arthroscopy is rarely required.

Ankle and Foot Fractures

See Table 6.4.

 HINTS AND TIPS

ANKLE AND FOOT FRACTURES

The Ottawa Ankle Rules provide guidelines as to when to x-ray the ankle, but whenever a bony injury is suspected a radiograph is required. Bi-malleolar fractures, tri-malleolar fractures and fractures with displacement (e.g. talar shift) indicate an unstable ankle injury that will likely require ORIF. Always assess clinically for an associated proximal fibular fracture (indicative of an unstable injury e.g. Maisonneuve injury) or a fracture of the 5th metatarsal base.

Achilles Tendon Rupture

A partial or full rupture of the Achilles tendon may occur and is frequently associated with sports.

Presentation

- Sudden onset of pain in the posterior aspect of the ankle and an inability to weight bear (partially or at all):
  - Passive ankle movement possible
- Simmonds/calf squeeze test is used to confirm rupture (see Chapter 2).

Investigations

- Ankle AP and lateral radiograph:
  - Indicated for suspected fracture
- USS calf:
  - Confirm diagnosis
  - Exclude a gastrocnemius muscle tear (pain often higher in midcalf).

Management

- Conservative:
  - Immobilization in equinus cast using a below-knee plaster or equivalent
  - Ten weeks of sequential casting routinely used then heel raise
- Surgical:
  - Indicated for recurrent injury
  - Evidence suggests no overall benefit over conservative management
  - Some advocate in athletes.

TABLE 6.4

THE SUBTYPES, PRESENTATION AND MANAGEMENT OF ANKLE AND FOOT FRACTURES

Management should always be tailored to the patients underlying co-morbidities and functional demands

Subtype	Presentation	Management (Complications)
Ankle	Indirect injury, e.g. inversion injury of ankle Associated medial ligament/bony injury and talar shift Fracture-dislocations do occur Assess for open injury and neurovascular status	(Postoperative, e.g. infection/ removal of metalwork, pain and stiffness, posttraumatic OA)
Weber A	Horizontal avulsion fibular fracture below syndesmosis	Immobilize in plaster/moonboot
Weber B	Spiral fibular fracture at syndesmosis, possible ligament damage (Figure 6.17)	Immobilize in plaster/moonboot if stable, ORIF considered for displacement and/or instability
Weber C	Fracture above syndesmosis, definite ligament damage	ORIF
Talus	Very rare and caused by a forced dorsiflexion High-energy trauma, e.g. RTA, fall from height Low-energy trauma, e.g. ankle sprain leading to avulsion Radiographs, with CT often required	ORIF for displacement or instability (Postoperative e.g. infection, AVN, OA)
Calcaneum	Fall onto heel, bilateral not uncommon High-energy trauma, e.g. fall from height Associated with spine, pelvis and tibial plateau injuries Radiographs, with CT often required	Elevation and immobilize non-weight bearing ORIF considered for notable displacement or instability (Postop, e.g. infection, deformity, OA, ACS, malunion)
Metatarsal*	Base fifth most common Inversion injury: avulsion due to action of peroneus brevis Other fractures by twisting or direct injury	Immobilize in plaster/moonboot ORIF for notable displacement/ multiple fractures (rare) (Pain, nonunion)

*A stress fracture of the second metatarsal is often called a 'march fracture'. It is often due to a repetitive low-intensity load that is applied to the bone. Further imaging is sometimes required and delayed union is not uncommon.

Complications

- Postoperative:
  - Infection, wound breakdown and neurovascular injury
- Recurrence of rupture.

Ankle Arthritis

Ankle arthritis is rarely idiopathic and is commonly secondary to trauma to the ankle joint, e.g. ankle fracture or tibial pilon fracture.

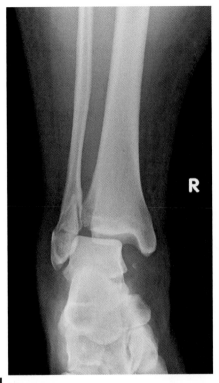

An AP radiograph of the right ankle demonstrating an unstable Weber B fracture of the lateral malleolus with medial joint space widening.

Presentation
- Progressive pain, swelling and stiffness of the ankle:
  - Reduced range of movement
- Associated deformities may be seen
- Previous scars, e.g. ORIF ankle.

Investigations
- AP and lateral standing of affected ankle
- MRI if concern re AVN.

Management
- Conservative:
  - Analgesia
  - Footwear modifications

- Surgical:
  - Fusion: for higher demand patients and deformity
  - Replacement: consider for older lower demand patients and minimal deformity.

Plantar Fasciitis

Plantar fasciitis is a self-limiting inflammation of the plantar fascia, which is often seen in middle-aged obese women. There is an association with Reiter disease (reactive arthritis). Bilateral symptoms do occur.

Presentation

- Heel pain, worse in the morning (after rest):
  - Radiates down foot
- Tenderness over the origin of the plantar fascia on the calcaneus (anteromedial aspect).
- Tight Achilles tendon leading to reduced range of ankle dorsiflexion.

Investigations

- Radiographs:
  - Rarely indicated but may show heel spur.

Management

- Conservative:
  - Analgesia, insoles, physiotherapy for stretching, and night immobilization
  - Local corticosteroid/anaesthetic injections
  - Shock wave therapy
- Surgical:
  - Release.

Hallux Valgus

 OVERVIEW

Hallux valgus is characterized by severe lateral deviation and rotation of the hallux, with medial deviation of the metatarsal (metatarsus primus varus). Pain and deformity are the common presenting features. Radiographs confirm the diagnosis. Conservative measures are the primary treatment, with surgery used for pain refractory to these measures.

Although primarily determined genetically (e.g. wide forefoot and varus big toe metatarsal), pain is exacerbated in people who chronically wear tight shoes or those with associated co-morbidities, e.g. RA, cerebral palsy, ligamentous laxity and pes planus. A medial bunion (metatarsal head and bursa hypertrophy) is common. It most frequently presents in women between 50 and 70 years of age.

Presentation

- Pain, tenderness, swelling and deformity of hallux:
  - Bunion that can be inflamed and irritated by footwear
  - Important to determine if fixed or flexible deformity
  - Metatarsalgia (pain across plantar metatarsal heads)
- Bilateral deformity

- Lesser toe deformities:
  - Second toe hammering
  - Assess for callosities and abnormal shoe wear pattern
- Assess for hindfoot and midfoot pathology:
  - Pes planus (see Chapter 2)
- Neurovascular status.

Investigations

- AP, lateral and oblique standing views of the feet:
  - Assess severity of deformity (intermetatarsal ankle and metatarsal phalangeal angle)

Management

- Conservative:
  - Footwear modifications including orthotics (moulded insoles)
- Surgical:
  - Indicated for symptoms (pain) and not cosmesis
  - Combination of soft tissue release and first metatarsal and proximal phalanx osteotomies, e.g. Scarf–Akin (common)
  - Lapidus procedure/fusion may be required for severe cases.

Complications

- Postoperative:
  - Infection and neurovascular injury
- Recurrence
- AVN
- OA
- Transfer metatarsalgia.

Hallux Rigidus

Hallux rigidus is arthritis affecting the MTPJ of the first ray. A history of trauma or microtrauma may be noted, but other causes should be considered, e.g. gout and inflammatory arthropathies.

Presentation

- Progressive pain, swelling and stiffness over the hallux MTPJ:
  - Pain worse on toe-off
- Reduced movement of hallux MTPJ:
  - Particularly in dorsiflexion secondary to dorsal osteophyte formation.

Investigations

- AP, lateral and oblique standing views of the feet.

Management

- Conservative:
  - Analgesia
  - Footwear modifications including orthotics (stiff-soled, deep toe box)
- Surgical:
  - Dorsal cheilectomy for isolated changes
  - Keller's procedure (excision of base of proximal phalanx) for low-demand elderly patients

- MTPJ fusion
- MTPJ replacement (debated).

Morton Neuroma

Morton neuroma is a compressive neuropathy and fibrosis of the interdigital nerves as they pass between the metatarsal heads. It is routinely seen in females (9:1). Repeated microtrauma from tight shoes is thought to exacerbate symptoms.

Presentation

- Most commonly affects second and third interdigital nerves
- Pain and paraesthesia in the affected web spaces
- Neuroma can sometimes be palpated between metatarsal heads
- Mulder click:
  - Squeeze metatarsal heads together (pain → metatarsalgia) but the test is positive if a click is heard in the affected web space.

Investigations

- AP, lateral and oblique standing views of the feet:
  - Rule out underlying structural/bony abnormality
- USS +/− injection:
  - Can confirm diagnosis but operator dependent.

Management

- Conservative:
  - Mainstay of treatment
  - Modified footwear (wide box shoe) and orthotics
  - Steroid injections (short-term benefit)
- Surgical:
  - Release and excision of the neuroma
  - Patient has a numb interdigital cleft.

Complications

- Postoperative:
  - Infection, neuroma and painful scar.

Tarsal Coalition

A congenital abnormality that leads to tarsal bone fusion, with the calcaneonavicular (8–12 yrs, most common) and talocalcaneal (12–15 yrs) most frequently affected.

Presentation

- Many are asymptomatic
- Pain exacerbated by activity:
  - Calf pain due to peroneal spasticity
- Deformities (see Chapter 2):
  - Assess standing
  - Pes planus (loss of normal medial arch)
  - Hindfoot valgus (check on tiptoe stance also)
  - Forefoot abduction (too many toes sign)
- Windlass test (see Chapter 2):
  - No medial arch forming on tiptoe stance = rigid flat foot.

Investigations

- AP, lateral and oblique radiographs of foot and ankle:
  - Harris view of calcaneum
- CT +/– MRI:
  - Confirm degree of coalition and any associated coalitions.

Management

- Conservative:
  - Symptomatic: commence with orthotics
- Surgical:
  - Resection of the coalition with interposition of fat or muscle
  - Subtalar/triple (subtalar, talonavicular, calcaneocuboid) arthrodesis in severe cases.

 HINTS AND TIPS

TARSAL COALITION

Pes planus (flat foot) can be a fixed (structural abnormality) or flexible deformity. The diagnosis can be confirmed on standing foot lateral radiographs. Other causes for pes planus include tibialis posterior tendon dysfunction, hindfoot and tarsometatarsal OA, and seronegative and inflammatory arthropathies. Pes cavus is defined by a high medial arch and is often associated with a varus hindfoot. This is often associated with neurological diseases, e.g. Charcot–Marie–Tooth disease, and a full neurological assessment is required. To determine if the deformity is fixed or rigid, the Coleman block test can be used.

HEAD, NECK AND SPINE

Head Injuries

 OVERVIEW

Head injuries are a common presentation to emergency departments. In most hospitals, if admission is necessary, these patients will be under the care of either the general or orthopaedic surgeons. All patients should have neurological observations and a low threshold now exists to proceed with CT head imaging when neurological symptoms or signs persist or progress.

Alcohol and assault are common coexisting factors with these patients, but it is important to remember that alcohol intoxication is not a sufficient reason for a deteriorating conscious level. The GCS is essential in the assessment and classification of these patients (Figure 6.18).

Presentation

Important aspects of the history are:

- Mode of injury, e.g. weapon used and blunt or penetrating injury
- Neurological symptoms, e.g. severe headache, persistent nausea and vomiting, seizure activity, amnesia and loss of consciousness
- Co-morbidities, e.g. alcohol excess and previous head injuries
- Current medications, in particular anticoagulation, e.g. warfarin.

Glasgow Coma Scale			
	Score		Score
Eye opening (*E*)		**Verbal response (*V*)**	
Spontaneous	4	Orientated	5
To speech	3	Confused conversation	4
To pain	2	Inappropriate words	3
No response	1	Incomprehensible sounds	2
		No response	1
Motor response (*M*)			
Obeys	6		
Localizes	5		
Withdraws (normal flexion)	4		
Abnormal flexion	3		
Extension	2		
No response	1		
Glasgow Coma Scale = *E* + *M* + *V*			
(GCS minimum = 3, maximum = 15, coma ≤ 8)			

FIGURE 6.18

Glasgow Coma Scale.

Examination should include:

- ABC
- Disability: general and neurological observations (GCS and pupils)
- Exposure: inspection for any external signs of trauma throughout the body
- Neurological exam to exclude any focal neurology and evidence of a skull fracture, e.g. Battle sign (retroauricular ecchymosis) or raccoon's eyes (periorbital ecchymosis) in a basal skull fracture, cerebrospinal fluid (CSF) leak (e.g. 'tram-lining' of nose-bleed discharge) and depressions
- A full general examination.

Investigations

- Alcohol reading and blood sugar
- Blood tests (e.g. sodium and glucose levels) and ECG where indicated
- Imaging:
  - Refer to guidelines
  - Skull X-ray and/or CT head:
    - Skull X-ray rarely used now
    - CT is the primary imaging modality when clinically indicated (refer to local and national guidelines)
  - A linear skull vault fracture increases the risk of an intracranial bleed by almost 400-fold.

Management (refer to local guidelines)

- ATLS guidelines should be followed initially, with particular importance placed on ABC and clearing the C-spine when neck injuries are suspected:
  - Ensure adequate cerebral perfusion and reduce intracranial pressure when elevated (normotonic i.v. fluids, mannitol, target low/normal pCO_2)
  - Intubation method and nasogastric tube placement:
    - Orogastric if basal skull fracture
- Admission should be considered in patients with:
  - GCS score that is less than 15 or fluctuating
  - Positive neurology, i.e. patients with persisting neurological symptoms (headache, nausea/vomiting, amnesia, irritability), seizure activity, or focal neurology on examination
  - Abnormal imaging
  - Inadequate social support or supervision
  - Risk of developing an intracranial bleed, e.g. patients on warfarin
- Regular neurological observations:
  - Those with persisting or worsening neurology should be considered for CT scanning
- Drugs:
  - Analgesia
  - Control bleeding and complete closure of open wounds
  - Avoid sedating drugs, e.g. diazepam for alcohol withdrawal
  - Tetanus and prophylactic antibiotics should be considered in open injuries
- Consider referral to neurosurgeons:
  - Intracranial lesion (diffuse brain injury, extradural/subdural/intracerebral haematomas) on imaging
  - Deteriorating or low GCS
  - Evolving neurology.

HINTS AND TIPS

HEAD INJURIES

All patients with a head injury must be assessed as per ATLS guidelines. It may not be possible to clinically clear the cervical spine in these patients and standard precautions should be maintained until this is possible. Always check the blood sugar level when assessing patients with a head injury, particularly with a history of alcohol excess. A low blood sugar level can be a missed reversible cause for a low GCS and must be excluded or treated for all patients.

Spinal Fractures

OVERVIEW

SPINAL FRACTURES

The acute management of all potential spinal injuries is airway with C-spine immobilization, followed by breathing, circulation and a full examination with log roll and PR examination (ATLS guidelines). The presence of a C-spine fracture

Continued

> **OVERVIEW—cont'd**
>
> increases the risk of fracture elsewhere in the spinal column. The vast majority of fractures are treated conservatively with immobilization. Surgical decompression and stabilization is recommended for neurology, severe displacement and instability. It is important to differentiate between neurogenic shock (hypotension, bradycardia) and spinal shock (transient areflexia below level of injury with loss of bulbocavernosus reflex).

Incomplete spinal cord injuries associated with spinal trauma can fit into the following categories:

- Anterior cord syndrome (flexion/rotation injuries) is paraplegia (legs more affected than arms) with loss of temperature and pain sensation.
- Central cord syndrome (e.g. syringomyelia) is motor loss in arms and legs (arms more affected than legs), with sacral sparing.
- Brown–Sequard syndrome is a hemisection of the cord with ipsilateral loss of power (paralysis) and proprioception, and loss of pain and temperature sensation on the contralateral side.
- Posterior cord syndrome (hyperextension injuries) is ataxia and loss of proprioception predominantly. Please see Table 6.5 for the presentation, investigation and management of specific spinal fractures.

> **HINTS AND TIPS**
>
> **SPINAL FRACTURES**
>
> When assessing spinal trauma or patients with back pain associated with red flag symptoms, plain radiographs of the spine can be used. They are of limited use in infection or malignancy as over 50% of bone destruction is required before this is detected. For imaging the soft tissues of the spine, persistent or progressive lower limb neurology, or suspected malignancy, MRI is the gold standard. CT is a useful tool in spinal trauma to assess the bony anatomy, and for other spinal pathologies when MRI is contraindicated.

Neck Pain

Neck pain is commonly seen in the elderly, but does not have the same magnitude of effect on young people as back pain. It is not commonly associated with significant spinal pathology, but may cause devastating quadriplegia in rare cases of cervical cord compression.

Causes

- Mechanical neck pain
- Acute neck sprain, i.e. whiplash
- Inflammation, e.g. RA
- Cervical myelopathy e.g. secondary to degenerative cervical disease
- Bone mineral disease, e.g. osteoporosis
- Cervical disc prolapse with radiculopathy
- Metastases
- Referred pain, e.g. from the diaphragm.

TABLE 6.5	
THE SUBTYPES, PRESENTATION AND MANAGEMENT OF SPINAL FRACTURES	
Steroids are recommended by some as an adjuvant in the management of acute spinal trauma	
Subtype	**Presentation, Investigations and Management**
Cervical	Types of injury: crush, burst, wedge fractures, facet joint dislocations
	Due to direct or indirect trauma; hyperflexion, extension or rotation
	Local tenderness, radiation to arms, associated head injury
	Neurological assessment, e.g. myotomes, dermatomes; C3-C5 keep the diaphragm alive
	Radiographs (AP/odontoid, lateral, C1-C7 and top T1; swimmer's view if needed). CT/MRI as required
C1	Atlas (Jefferson) burst fracture, direct load to top of head
C2	Type 1, 2 or 3 odontoid fracture; hangman's posterior fracture (spondylolisthesis C2/3)
C5-C6	Common position for fracture and/or subluxation
	Treatment ranges from immobilization to fixation for displacement/instability; joint fusion for nonunion
Thoracic	Types of injury: crush, burst, wedge fractures, T11-L1 thoracolumbar dislocation
	Due to direct or indirect trauma; hyperflexion, extension or rotation
	Pathological bone, e.g. osteoporotic
	Local tenderness, paraplegia if unstable/displaced, associated head injury
	Full neurological assessment, e.g. myotomes, dermatomes
	Radiographs (AP, lateral). CT/MRI as required
	Treatment is with immobilization; fixation for instability/neurology/pathological fractures
Lumbar	Types of injury: compression or transverse process fractures
	Pathological bone, e.g. osteoporotic
	Local tenderness, cauda equina syndrome if displaced (see spinal cord compression)
	Full neurological assessment, e.g. myotomes, dermatomes, saddle anaesthesia, per rectum examination
	Radiographs (AP, lateral). CT/MRI as required
	Treatment is with immobilization; fixation for instability, neurology or pathological fractures

Presentation

- Acute asymmetrical decreased ROM of neck
- History of trauma or persistent uncomfortable posture
- Assess for direct spinal tenderness
- Pain from the neck may radiate to:
  - Head: temple, occiput or face
  - Upper limb: scapula, shoulder or upper arm
- Radicular pain and neurological symptoms:
  - C6 compression common
  - C7 or C8 compression less common.

Investigations

- As for back pain.

Management

- Conservative measures in majority of cases
- Surgery (decompression +/– spinal fusion):
  - Indicated for severe neurological presentations, e.g. progressive cervical myelopathy or persistent debilitating radicular pain/weakness.

Lumbar Back Pain

 OVERVIEW

> Lumbar back pain is a collective term for a group of conditions that present with this exceedingly common complaint. It is essential to exclude progressive neurological and red flag signs when assessing such patients. Bloods and MRI are indicated when sinister pathology is suspected.

It is reported that approximately 30% of UK homes have one adult or more who is in pain, with 25% of these households having two adults in that position. Back pain is an important cause of absenteeism from work and the cost of managing back pain and sciatica alone is approximately £12.3 billion/year.

Causes

See Figure 6.19.

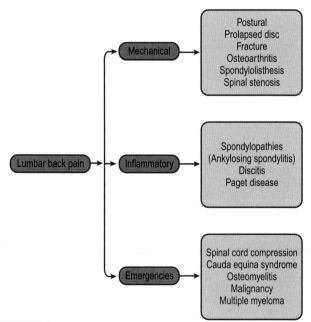

FIGURE 6.19

Classification of causes of lumbar back pain.

Presentation

- The presentation of mechanical and inflammatory conditions is somewhat similar. Important differentiating factors are as follows:
  - Age at onset:
    - <50 years: mechanical postural pain, prolapsed disc and spondylopathies
    - >50 years: degenerative condition, osteoporosis and malignancy
  - Rate of onset and the time of day the pain is most notable
  - Unilateral or bilateral back and leg pain
  - The presence of morning stiffness and the effect of exercise
  - Remember red flag signs (Chapter 2):
    - Neurological symptoms and signs
    - Bladder, bowel or sexual dysfunction.

Investigations

- Blood tests including:
  - CRP/ESR which may be increased in inflammatory back pain or infection
  - Bone screen for multiple myeloma, Paget disease, etc.
  - Prostate specific antigen if presentation suggests prostatic disease
- Radiographs: disc space narrowing and joint arthritis
- MRI: indicated for neurological deficits and malignancy
- CT and bone scan: spondylolisthesis, some bone tumours, e.g. osteoid osteoma, and where MRI is contraindicated.

Management

- Conservative for most:
  - Almost 90% resolve within 6 weeks of onset
  - Analgesics, e.g. NSAIDs
  - Limited bed rest, though dependent on cause
  - Physiotherapy
- Surgical:
  - Root-cause dependent
  - Caudal or facet joint injections advocated by some
  - Spinal decompression +/− fusion.

Prolapsed Intervertebral Disc

Prolapse involves nerve root compression due to posterolateral herniation of the nucleus pulposus through the annulus fibrosus, with a predisposition for the L4-L5 and L5-S1 regions. It is reported to affect 2–5% of the population and is associated with males aged 30–50 years, long-distance drivers, heavy manual labourers, smoking and socioeconomic deprivation.

Presentation

- Back pain, referred leg pain and sciatica
- Motor and/or sensory symptoms and signs over the distribution of the nerve root being irritated:
  - Paraesthesia, weakness and absent reflexes of affected nerve root(s)
- Higher disc prolapses may affect the femoral nerve instead
- Exacerbating factors are sitting, coughing and sneezing
- Straight leg raise test may be positive for nerve root irritation.

Investigation
- MRI.

Management
- Conservative:
  - Involves initial rest (avoid prolonged), analgesia and physiotherapy
  - Nerve root steroid injections advocated by some
- Surgery:
  - Microdiscectomy (endoscopic, miniopen), open discectomy.

 HINTS AND TIPS

PROLAPSED INTERVERTEBRAL DISC

Conservative measures such as analgesia and physiotherapy will result in 70–90% of patients experiencing resolution or improvement of symptoms within 3 months of onset. Recurrence is possible and patients need to be advised regarding this.

Spinal Cord Compression

Acute spinal cord compression is an emergency and may be associated with a variety of causes:

- Tumour (local or metastatic):
  - 98% of spinal tumours are metastases
- Abscess, e.g. epidural abscess, cold abscess of tuberculosis
- Trauma
- Disc prolapse (central)

Presentation
- Assess for red flag symptoms
- Bilateral progressive leg +/− back pain is common
- Radicular (nerve root) pain at the compression level
- Paraesthesia below the compression level
- Upper and lower motor neurone signs dependent on the compression level:
  - Upper motor neurone: increased tone/spasticity, hyperreflexia, muscle spasms and weakness, disuse atrophy, positive Hoffman sign, clonus and upgoing plantar response
  - Lower motor neurone lesion: decreased tone/flaccidity, hyporeflexia, fasciculation, motor weakness and severe atrophy, sensory loss and down going plantar response
- Sphincter disturbance
- Cauda equina syndrome indicates lumbar (L1 and below central lumbar disc) nerve root compression and results in characteristic lower motor neurone symptoms:
  - Micturition disturbance with key features of hesitancy, urgency, painless retention and eventual overflow incontinence
  - Faecal incontinence due to anal sphincter tone dysfunction
  - Increasing motor weakness associated with gait disorder
  - Saddle (perianal) anaesthesia.

Investigations
- Blood tests:
  - FBC, UEs, LFTs
  - Inflammatory markers
  - Prostate specific antigen if indicated
  - TFTs and serum B_{12}
- Lumbar puncture if not contraindicated
- Chest and plain spinal radiographs:
  - Vertebral collapse or erosions
- CT and bone scan +/– biopsy
- Spinal MRI.

Management

Treatment is determined by the cause and location of the lesion. The common therapeutic options are:

- Analgesia
- High-dose i.v. corticosteroids, e.g. dexamethasone 8–16mg
- Bisphosphonates
- Urgent surgical exploration with decompression or excision and stabilization
- Chemotherapy or radiotherapy for malignant disease.

 HINTS AND TIPS

SPINAL CORD COMPRESSION

Cauda equina syndrome accounts for 2–6% of all lumbar disc herniations and most commonly presents in men between 20 and 45 years of age, secondary to a large central disc prolapse at the L4-L5 level. The presence of unilateral signs and the absence of pain do not exclude the diagnosis and urgent MRI is indicated for suspected cases. Urgent decompression in confirmed cases is required.

Spondylolisthesis

 OVERVIEW

Spondylolisthesis is a forward translation (slip) of one vertebral body on the one below. It may be associated with certain sports that involve repetitive hyperextension of the spine and it is important to assess for associated neurology and whether this is evolving. Decompression and fusion is required for severe slips.

One of the common causes of a spondylolisthesis is a defect of the pars interarticularis (ossification defect), with a predisposition for the L4-L5 and L5-S1 levels. A pars defect without slip is more common and is known as spondylolysis. This usually occurs in Caucasians, males, children and athletes (gymnasts), and is associated with other spinal pathologies (scoliosis, kyphosis).

Presentation
- Chronic back pain on standing and exercise
- Exacerbating factor is spinal hyperextension

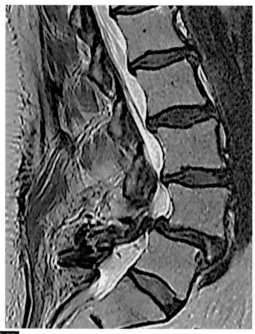

FIGURE 6.20
An MRI sagittal section with an L4-L5 spondylolisthesis.

- Movement and exercise sometimes restricted
- Sciatica and radiculopathy are common.

Investigation

- Radiographs:
  - 'Scottie dog' sign
- CT and/or MRI (Figure 6.20)
- Wiltse classification:
  - Congenital, isthmic (pars lesion), degenerative, traumatic, pathological and postsurgical
- Myerding classification (slip severity):
  - Type 1 = <25%, type 2 = 25–50%, type 3 = 51–75%, type 4 = 76–100%, and type 5 = >100% (spondyloptosis).

Management

- Conservative:
  - Rest (avoid prolonged), analgesia and physiotherapy
- Surgery:
  - Decompression and spinal fusion is indicated for severe slips.

Spinal Stenosis

Stenosis (narrowing) of the spinal canal is most commonly due to degenerative changes (facet joint hypertrophy/cyst, ligamentum flavum hypertrophy) presenting between 50 and 70 years of age. It is less commonly associated with disc prolapse, inflammation (e.g. ankylosing spondylitis), malignancy or congenital narrowing (e.g. achondroplasia). Narrowing of the canal and foramen can lead to neural compression and ischaemia, resulting in the classical symptoms described below.

Presentation

- Exacerbating factors are exercise and spinal extension, e.g. standing or walking, leading to back pain referred to the buttocks and legs (spinal or neurogenic claudication)
  - Relief is achieved by spinal flexion and rest
- Nerve root compression leading to neurological symptoms
- Cauda equina is rare.

Investigations

- CT or MRI to confirm:
  - AP diameter or cross-sectional area assessed
- Remember to exclude vascular causes (peripheral vascular disease).

Management

- Conservative:
  - Lifestyle changes (weight loss), analgesia and physiotherapy
- Surgery:
  - Required in approximately a third of cases
  - Decompression +/− fusion.

 HINTS AND TIPS

SPINAL STENOSIS

The key diagnosis is differentiating symptoms and signs of spinal claudication from those of vascular claudication. Both will lead to pain on exercise; however, vascular claudication will resolve with standing still, but spinal flexion (i.e. leaning forward) is needed to relieve spinal claudication. Distal pulses are routinely intact in the spinal claudication patient, unless they have concomitant peripheral vascular disease.

Scoliosis

Scoliosis is a 3D coronal lateral curvature of the thoracolumbar spine with rotational deformity of the vertebrae and ribs. The classification of scoliosis can be defined as:

- Postural: secondary to a pathology outwith the spine causing a mild scoliosis that is often seen in children and with pelvic obliquity, and where bending forward abolishes the curve.
- Structural: a fixed deformity from within the spine that does not change with posture.

The causes of scoliosis are:

- Congenital or infantile: irregularity leading to atypical spinal development, e.g. hemi-vertebrae and osteopathic scoliosis
- Idiopathic: cause is unknown, e.g. adolescent idiopathic scoliosis
- Neurological: neuromuscular abnormality leads to uneven forces on the spine, e.g. cerebral palsy
- Secondary: rare primary cause leads to secondary curvature of the spine, e.g. leg length discrepancy and hip deformity
- Degenerative: usually of the lumbar spine in the elderly.

Adolescent Idiopathic Scoliosis

Adolescent idiopathic scoliosis is commonly seen before puberty, and ceases when growth comes to an end. It is typically characterized by lateral curvature of the thoracolumbar spine (>10°), with rotational deformity of the vertebrae and ribs (convex to right) causing a prominent hump on spine flexion. A right thoracic curve is most commonly seen and it is more frequent in girls, who are usually tall for their age.

Known risk factors for increasing progression of the curve are: girls, more growth is expected, rate at which the curve and growth are occurring, and curve type (thoracic > lumbar, double > single) and degree.

Presentation

- Peripubertal girls commonly but not exclusively
- Spinal curve often first seen by parents
- One shoulder elevated above the other
- Decreased chest expansion
- Neurological examination:
  - Abdominal reflexes.

Investigations

- Radiographs (full PA and lateral standing of spine, Figure 6.21):
  - Right thoracic curve most common
  - Cobb angle is the maximum angle of curvature of the primary curve (greater than 10° is diagnostic)
  - Lenke or King classifications
  - Risser staging: assessment of closure of epiphyseal growth plates of iliac apophysis to assess skeletal maturity
- MRI.

Management

Dependent on the size of the curve and the age/maturity of the patient, i.e. possible progression, as most curves should not progress beyond skeletal maturity. Options include:

- Conservative:
  - Observation with surveillance radiographs (curve <25°)
  - Bracing to limit progression for flexible 25–40° curves (does not correct)

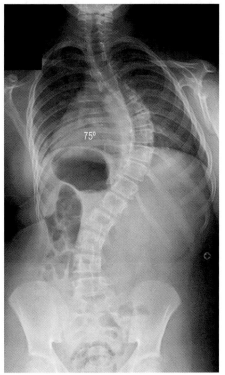

FIGURE 6.21

Adolescent idiopathic scoliosis with a 75° right thoracic curve.

- Surgical:
  - Indicated for severely progressing curves (>40–45°) and trunk imbalance
  - Anterior and/or posterior (most common) spinal fusion
  - Continuous spinal cord monitoring intraoperatively.

 HINTS AND TIPS

SCOLIOSIS

MRI can be necessary for preoperative planning but may also be required to exclude associated intraspinal anomalies, e.g. syrinx or tethered cord.

BONE AND JOINT INFECTIONS

 OVERVIEW

This section covers the management of bone and joint infections in both children and adults. A combination of clinical assessment, blood tests (including inflammatory markers), radiological imaging and microbiology results are used in the diagnosis of bone and joint infection. Although inflammatory markers are useful, they are not specific for infection, and the ESR can be normal in the acute phase. Plain radiographs normally only detect significant and chronic bone destruction or prosthetic loosening. Ultrasound can be useful in children to look for joint and soft tissue collections, but also to confirm any periosteal reaction indicative of osteomyelitis, with guided aspiration or biopsy possible. MRI is seen by many as the gold standard in the diagnosis of bone and joint infection. Management is with source control when required and a prolonged course of antibiotic therapy. Surgery is usually for abscess drainage and chronic infection.

Septic Arthritis

Septic arthritis occurs when there is a bacterial infection of the joint. It is a surgical emergency. Untreated septic arthritis can lead rapidly (within hours) to life-threatening sepsis, as well as cause joint destruction due to release of proteolytic enzymes that degrade bone, cartilage and soft tissues. The incidence is 2–10/100 000 but septic arthritis is more common in patients with arthroplasty and coexisting joint diseases such as RA. Joints of the lower limb are most frequently affected and the hip (most common in infants) and knee (most common in children and adults) are the commonest sites. However, any joint, and sometimes more than one joint, can be affected.

Pathogenesis

The disease usually occurs as the result of bacterial spread from another site. The most common primary sites of infection are:

- The skin, possibly compromised due to trauma, e.g. cellulitis or surgery
- Neighbouring bone (e.g. in osteomyelitis, uncommon in the knee as the metaphysis is extra-articular)
- Haematogenous spread (e.g. respiratory or urinary tract infection).

The organisms most commonly implicated include (Table 6.6):

- *Staphylococcus aureus* (most common)
- Gram-negative bacilli (e.g. elderly, diabetics, immunocompromised)
- *Neisseria gonorrhoeae* (sexually transmitted infection in adults)
- *Haemophilus influenzae* (nonimmunized neonates and infants)
- *Staphylococcus epidermidis* (joint replacements).

Risk factors include:

- Extremes of age
- Socioeconomic deprivation
- Preexisting joint disease, e.g. RA
- Preexisting sepsis, i.e. haematogenous spread

TABLE 6.6

CAUSATIVE ORGANISMS FOR BONE AND JOINT INFECTIONS

Type	Organisms	Common Clinical Scenario
Gram positive	*Staphylococcus aureus*	Most common for all case types
	Coagulase-negative staphylococci:	Prosthetic infection
	• *Staphylococcus epidermidis*	
	Streptococcus pneumoniae	
	Beta-haemolytic streptococci	
	Streptococcus viridans	Prosthetic infection
Gram negative	Enterobacteriaceae:	
	• *Escherichia coli*	Extremes of age
	• *Klebsiella*	
	• *Salmonella*	Sickle cell patients
	Pseudomonas	
	Haemophilus	Nonimmunized children
	Neisseria gonorrhoeae	Sexually transmitted infections
Others	Anaerobes	
	Fungi	Immunocompromised patients
	Mycobacterium tuberculosis	

Adapted from Table 40.1 in Datta PK, Bulstrode CJK, Nixon IJ. MCQs and EMQs in Surgery: A Bailey & Love Revision Guide. 2nd edition. CRC Press; 2015.

- Immunosuppression, e.g. diabetes, HIV/AIDS, steroids and intravenous drug use
- Diabetes mellitus.

Presentation

- Acute onset of a painful, red, hot and swollen joint
- Muscle spasm leading to immobility of joint (pseudoparesis)
- Systemic upset: tachycardia, fever and malaise
- Atypical presentation may occur in the elderly, the immunosuppressed or those with established joint disease
- Polyarthralgia, tenosynovitis, urogenital symptoms and a pustular rash may occur in *N. gonorrhoeae* infection
- Chronic infection in a total joint replacement may result in loosening of the implant. This may be the sole clinical feature of infection.

Investigations

- Blood tests:
  - Haematology: raised ESR and WCC
  - Biochemistry: raised CRP
- Joint aspiration before antibiotics given (see Chapter 3, Table 3.3):
  - Turbid fluid/pus with raised WCC
  - Organism may be demonstrated by urgent microscopy and Gram staining or isolated by culture
- Microbiology:
  - Obtain blood cultures and/or cultures from possible sites of primary infection (wound site, urogenital system, chest)

- Imaging:
  - Radiographs: joint effusion and soft tissue swelling
  - USS: presence of effusion and may aid diagnostic aspiration; good first line in children
  - MRI has a high sensitivity and specificity but often not required.

Management

- Resuscitation as necessary and high-dose intravenous antibiotics:
  - Empirical then targeted (microbiology) for 1–2 weeks or more, followed by oral therapy (total duration or treatment ~6–12 weeks but case dependent)
- Analgesia
- Surgery:
  - Joint incision and drainage with lavage is the gold standard
  - Repeated joint aspiration or washout may be required
  - Removal of infected implant material (see Hip and Knee Arthroplasty section in this chapter).

Prognosis

The prognosis is good with appropriate early treatment but complications may occur including:

- Septic shock
- Abscess or sinus formation
- Joint destruction, periarticular osteoporosis, ankylosis and secondary OA
- Avascular necrosis
- Inhibition of limb growth and deformity (with growth plate involvement in children).

 HINTS AND TIPS

SEPTIC ARTHRITIS

The most common cause of native and prosthetic joint infections is a Gram positive organism, with *S. aureus* frequently the causative organism. For a prosthetic infection a coagulase-negative staphylococci (normal skin commensal) may be seen. For the effective management of joint infection, it is paramount to identify the causative organism, or even the combination of organisms, which are responsible. Although early empirical intravenous antibiotics are essential in the presence of life-threatening sepsis, it is advised that multiple microbiological samples are collected prior to this when possible. In the presence of sepsis, blood cultures and joint aspiration can quickly be performed prior to administration of antibiotics.

Acute Osteomyelitis

Osteomyelitis is infection of the bone. In children it commonly occurs at the metaphysis close to the epiphyseal plate whereas in adults any site in the bone may be affected.

Pathogenesis

Spread of infection to bone occurs via: (1) blood-borne spread from the skin or respiratory, gastrointestinal or genitourinary tract; or (2) direct spread posttrauma (including surgery). Common infecting organisms include (Table 6.6):

- *S. aureus*
- *Streptococcus pneumoniae* or *Streptococcus pyogenes*
- Salmonella (associated with patients who have sickle cell disease)
- *H. influenzae* and haemolytic streptococci (children).

Risk factors include:

- Extremes of age
- Immunosuppression (e.g. HIV, AIDS, steroids, intravenous drug use)
- Diabetes mellitus
- Joint replacement
- Trauma.

Presentation

- Pain, tenderness, warmth and redness over affected bone
- Loss of function (e.g. unable to weight bear, particularly in children)
- Vertebrae can be affected
- Effusion of nearby joint(s)
- Systemic upset: fever, malaise, anorexia and weight loss.

Investigations

- Blood tests:
  - Haematology: raised ESR and WCC
  - Biochemistry: raised CRP
- Microbiology:
  - Culture of affected site if indicated/possible
  - Blood cultures or culture from site of primary infection (e.g. skin, wound, urogenital tract) before antibiotics given
- Imaging:
  - Radiographs initially normal, but within weeks changes can include osteolysis, metaphyseal rarefaction, and subsequently periosteal elevation and bone formation, and osteosclerosis and cortical thickening are possible
  - USS: presence of periosteal reaction; is a good first line in children
  - CT and MRI.

Management

- Resuscitation as necessary and high-dose intravenous antibiotics:
  - Empirical then targeted (microbiology) for 1–2 weeks or more, followed by oral therapy (total duration or treatment ~6–12 weeks as but case dependent)
- Rest analgesia in acute phase but early mobilization when possible
- Nonpharmacological approaches:
  - Initial rest and then mobilization with physiotherapy as required
- Surgery:
  - Surgical drainage with removal of metalwork, dead bone and tissue as indicated.

Prognosis

Good with appropriate treatment but several complications may occur including:

- Septic arthritis
- Bone deformity and growth disturbance
- Fracture (pathological)
- Chronic osteomyelitis and/or recurrence
- Abscess formation:
  - Brodie abscess (Figure 6.22) is a less severe form of osteomyelitis where natural defences have partially overcome the infection, leading to an abscess confined within cortical/sclerotic bone (in the metaphysis). This appears as a halo on MRI. This type of abscess is commonly associated with distal femoral and tibial injuries.

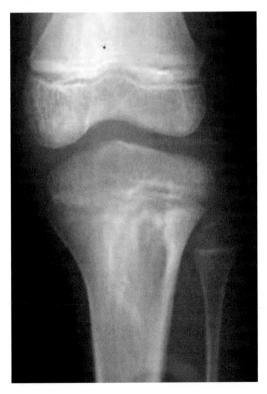

FIGURE 6.22

A Brodie abscess of the proximal tibia.

HINTS AND TIPS

ACUTE OSTEOMYELITIS

In children acute osteomyelitis occurs more commonly through haematogenous spread, whereas in adults it frequently occurs secondary to direct inoculation, e.g. after open fracture. CT can be used for infected nonunions following fracture and may aid in diagnosing the presence of sequestra. MRI again is the gold standard. Isotope bone scanning is sensitive, but nonspecific.

Chronic Osteomyelitis

Chronic osteomyelitis is a persistent bone infection that sometimes follows acute osteomyelitis (due to persistent infection/poor antibiotic delivery to necrotic bone or antibiotic-resistant microorganisms), particularly in patients with prosthetic implants or those with metalwork in place after (open) fracture fixation.

Initial infection and inflammation of the metaphysis lead to lifting and removal of the periosteum due to a subperiosteal abscess, leading eventually to original bone death (sequestrum) due to a compromised blood supply causing necrosis (cortex infarction), with new bone formation as a consequence (involucrum). The Cierny–Mader classification can be used for chronic osteomyelitis, with an aim to try to guide management and be prognostic of the outcome. The groups are:

1. Medullary
2. Superficial
3. Localized
4. Diffuse.

Presentation
- Pain, swelling and redness over affected site (e.g. long bones)
- Sinus, ulcer or abscess development
- Systemic upset, weight loss and fever
- Risk factors are similar to those for acute osteomyelitis.

Investigations
- Blood tests:
  - Haematology: raised ESR and WCC
  - Biochemistry: raised CRP
- Microbiology:
  - Blood cultures and cultures from affected site or likely primary site (a bone biopsy may be needed)
- Imaging:
  - Radiographs show osteosclerosis, cortical thickening, sequestrum, periosteal reaction and areas of osteolysis
  - CT and/or MRI will help differentiate soft tissue infection and necrotic bone.

Management

- Long-term antibiotic treatment, choice is culture-dependent
- Pain relief with analgesics
- Lifestyle changes, e.g. stop smoking and NSAIDs, and better nutrition
- Surgery:
  - Drainage with dead bone removal and external fixation, e.g. Ilizarov technique
  - Removal of implants or metalwork
  - Amputation can be rarely indicated.

Prognosis

Various complications may occur including:

- Pathological fracture
- Secondary amyloidosis
- Squamous cell carcinoma of sinus and surrounding skin (Marjolin ulcer).

 HINTS AND TIPS

CHRONIC OSTEOMYELITIS

NSAIDs should be avoided in the presence of nonunion, as they are known to delay bone healing. A long-standing sinus associated with chronic osteomyelitis can rarely result in a Marjolin ulcer. This requires a wide surgical excision, or even sometimes amputation, with recurrence rates 20–50%.

Viral Arthritis

Viral infection may be associated with an acute, but self-limiting, form of arthritis. Viruses that have been implicated include:

- Hepatitis B and C
- HIV (also can be associated with chronic polyarthralgia)
- Chickenpox
- Mumps
- Erythrovirus (formerly parvovirus) B19
- Rubella.

Presentation

- Acute polyarthritis with a variable distribution
- History of recent 'viral' illness
- Fever or rash.

Investigations

- Microbiology:
  - IgM antibodies to offending pathogen on serological testing.

Management

- NSAIDs/analgesics
- Most cases are self-limiting.

MUSCULOSKELETAL TUMOURS

 OVERVIEW

Benign tumours of the bone include osteoid osteoma, osteochondroma, enchondromas and giant cell tumour. Malignant tumours of the bone include myeloma (most common primary malignant bone tumour), osteosarcoma (most common malignant primary bone sarcoma), Ewing sarcoma, chondrosarcoma and secondary bone tumours. Metastases are the most commonly seen malignant bone tumours. As in bone tumours, soft tissue tumours can be benign, e.g. a simple lipoma, or malignant, e.g. liposarcoma. Biopsy provides the definitive diagnosis.

Classification, Assessment and Management

The benign and malignant Enneking classifications for bone tumours are most frequently used, although the related TNM staging system is often used in clinical practice. The benign classification divides tumours into:

- Latent: can be asymptomatic, e.g. enchondroma.
- Active: minimal symptoms and routinely slow growing, e.g. unicameral bone cyst.
- Aggressive: often symptomatic and can grow very quickly, e.g. giant cell tumour of bone.

Malignant tumours are classified according to grade (1 = low grade, 2 = high grade), whether the tumour extends beyond the bone cortices (A = intracompartmental, B = extracompartmental) and whether there are associated metastases (stage 3). The most common presentation for bone tumours is an Enneking stage 2B.

SOFT TISSUE TUMOURS. When assessing soft tissue tumours, there are some generally agreed criteria for a lump that may be sinister and requires further investigation. Many advocate that any lesion greater than the size of a golf ball requires a diagnosis. Important symptoms and signs are pain, increasing in size, larger than 5 cm, recurrence of lump at previous excision site and deep to the fascia, i.e. not superficial.

PATHOLOGICAL FRACTURES. The Mirel's pathological fracture scoring system is used to stratify the risk of a pathological fracture of a bony metastasis. It includes four categories (tumour, pain, lesion, size) that are scored on a scale of 1–3 (Table 6.7). With a score of ≤7 the fracture risk is <5% and prophylactic fixation is not considered to be indicated. For a score of 8, clinical judgement on a case-by-case basis is required as the fracture risk is ~15–30%. For a score ≥9, prophylactic fixation is indicated with fracture risk 30–100%.

Routine Investigations

The routine workup for a suspected bone or soft tissue tumour will often include:

TABLE 6.7		
THE MIRELS SCORING SYSTEM FOR PATHOLOGICAL FRACTURE RISK ASSESSMENT		
Category	**Scoring**	**Description**
Tumour	1	Upper limb
	2	Lower limb
	3	Peritrochanteric/proximal femur
Pain	1	Mild
	2	Moderate
	3	Severe/functional
Lesion	1	Blastic
	2	Mixed
	3	Lytic
Size	1	<1/3 of cortical thickness
	2	1/3–2/3 cortical thickness
	3	>2/3 cortical thickness

- Plain radiographs or USS for soft tissue lesions
- MRI +/− biopsy
- Staging CT if malignancy confirmed
- Bloods including a bone profile.

Management

A biopsy will provide the definitive diagnosis and determine further management which can include a combination of surgical excision, chemotherapy, radiotherapy and palliative care. Adequacy of surgical resection of a tumour is assessed by depth of the resection margins. Intralesional resection is defined as a margin through the lesion. Marginal resection is defined as through the reactive zone of the tumour, with a wide excision outside the reactive zone. A radical resection is the excision of the whole compartment.

Osteoid Osteoma

Osteoid osteoma is a benign bone-forming tumour of young males, often localizing to the diaphysis of the major long bones, the femoral neck and spine. It is most common between the ages of 5 and 30 years. The clinical and histological presentation of an osteoblastoma is similar.

Presentation

- Severe dull pain
- Often worse at night and not related to activity
- Classically relieved by NSAIDs.

Investigation

- Radiographs of affected limb/area:
  - Sclerosis with a radiolucent nidus
  - If tumour >2 cm it is routinely defined as an osteoblastoma
- CT +/− bone scan.

Management

- Observation and NSAIDs
- Surgical excision or ablation if prominent/persistent symptoms are present.

Osteochondroma

Osteochondroma is a very common benign cartilage tumour of children and adolescents, often localizing to the metaphyses of the major long bones. It forms from anomalous cartilage found on the outer surface of the growth plate; endochondral ossification under the cartilage may result in sessile (flattened) or pedunculated (stalked) bony lesions covered with hyaline cartilage. An autosomal dominant multiple form exists: multiple osteochondromatosis (MO) or multiple hereditary exostosis (MHE) (Figure 6.23). Malignant transformation is infrequent.

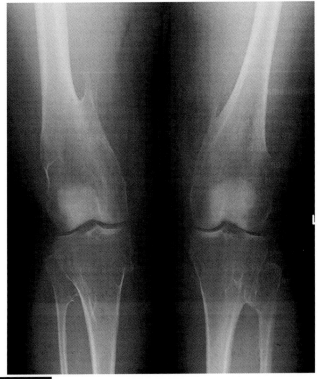

FIGURE 6.23
MO of both knees.

Presentation

- Most give minimal symptoms
- If symptomatic it is often due to compression/irritation of adjacent soft tissue structures.

Investigation

- Radiographs of affected limb/area:
  - Bony outgrowth stalk with a classic 'mushroom' type appearance.
- CT +/– MRI:
  - Assess for sinister features and preoperative planning if adjacent to neurovasculature.

Management

- Excision indicated only if prominent symptoms are present.

 HINTS AND TIPS

OSTEOCHONDROMA

MO is an autosomal dominant condition where multiple osteochondromas/exostosis occur, potentially leading to deformities of the skeleton, e.g. bowing of the forearm and radial head dislocation. It is associated with mutation in one of the EXT genes. Malignant change to chondrosarcoma is infrequent in solitary lesions, with a 2–4% lifetime risk in MO.

Enchondroma

Enchondroma is a common benign hyaline cartilage tumour routinely found in adults commonly between 20 and 50 years of age. Areas affected include the medullary cavity within the metaphysis of long bones, e.g. femur, but also within the small bones of the hand and feet.

Presentation

- Most are asymptomatic unless impending or actual pathological fracture
- Pain, swelling and deformity may occur due to large tumours

Investigation

- Radiographs of affected limb/area:
  - Scalloped oval lucent/lytic regions, patchy calcification.

Management

- Curettage indicated only if prominent symptoms or with pathological fracture.

 HINTS AND TIPS

ENCHONDROMA

Surveillance radiographs are necessary to confirm no malignant transformation. Two multiple forms of enchondroma include Ollier's disease (associated with skeletal dysplasia and long bone deformity) which has a risk of malignant transformation of 20–30%, and Maffucci's syndrome (associated with soft tissue angiomas) where the risk of malignant transformation is up to 100%.

Giant Cell Tumours

Giant cell tumours (osteoclastomas) are locally aggressive (benign Enneking stage 3) and potentially recurrent tumours of young adults (20–40 years), often localizing to the epiphysis of long bones, particularly around the knee and distal radius. Lung metastases are very rare (<1–5%).

Presentation

- Pain and loss of motion of the affected joint.

Investigation

- Radiographs of affected limb/area:
  - Nonsclerotic, expanding lytic/cystic lesions, extend to subchondral region, 'soap bubble' appearance
- MRI with bone biopsy
- CXR and CT chest are used to detect metastases.

Management

Radical curettage +/– adjuvant treatment (e.g. phenol or hydrogen peroxide) +/– reconstruction.

Multiple Myeloma

Myeloma is the most frequently seen primary bone tumour, arising from the proliferation of plasma cells (B cells) in the bone marrow. It is often seen in those aged >50 years, peaking at 65–70 years, and is more common in males. Multiple myeloma with widespread metastases is common, although single lesions (plasmacytoma) do occur but often progress.

Presentation

- Can mimic metastases with unknown primary
- Pain of site affected, e.g. ribs or spine
- Pathological fracture
- Anaemia or renal failure
- Infection.

Investigation

- Bloods: ↓Hb, ↑ESR, ↑Ca^{2+}, ↑immunoglobulin plasma protein electrophoresis, urea and creatinine
- Urine: Bence-Jones protein and ↑immunoglobulin protein electrophoresis
- Radiographs of affected limb/area:
  - Punched-out lesions (Figure 6.24)
- MRI and a bone marrow biopsy.

Management

- Bone marrow transplant +/– chemotherapy
- Median term survival: 3–5 years
- Otherwise symptomatic management:
  - Bisphosphonates, radiotherapy and fixation (bone pain/fracture)
  - Erythropoietin +/– transfusion (anaemia)
  - Dialysis (renal failure).

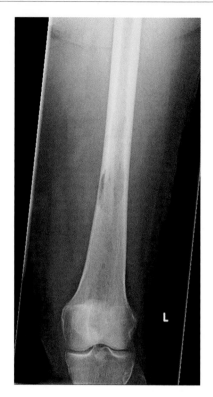

FIGURE 6.24

A myeloma deposit in the left distal femur.

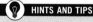

> **HINTS AND TIPS**
>
> **MULTIPLE MYELOMA**
>
> A bone scan can be negative (cold) with multiple myeloma. Bone marrow transplant with chemotherapy is the only curative option.

Osteosarcoma

Osteosarcoma is a very rare, but the most common, malignant bone tumour of children and older adults (bi-modal age distribution), particularly males (~1.5 : 1). It is associated with retinoblastoma, Paget's disease and radiation. Localization is often in the metaphyses of the long bones (e.g. femur, tibia, humerus), often leading to bone destruction. Blood-borne metastases may occur in the lung.

Presentation
- Bone pain, swelling and sometimes erythema
- Usually a mass felt
- Respiratory symptoms, e.g. cough or shortness of breath, if lung metastases.

Investigations
- Bloods: ↑ESR, ↑ALP
- Radiographs:
  - Lytic sclerosis, Codman triangle (periosteal reaction), sunray spicules and bone destruction
- MRI and bone biopsy

Management
- Neo-adjuvant and postoperative multiagent chemotherapy
- Subsequent excision and reconstruction:
  - Amputation is possible
- Five-year survival of approximately 60–80% with modern treatment.

Ewing's Sarcoma

Ewing's sarcoma is a very rare, but extremely malignant, small round cell bone tumour of children and young adults (5–25 years of age). Localization is usually in the diaphysis of long and flat bones, e.g. femur, pelvis or spine, frequently leading to bone destruction. Blood-borne metastases often occur to the lung, liver and other parts of the skeleton.

Presentation
- Bone pain, swelling and tenderness
- Possibly with fever and anaemia (can mimic infection).

Investigations
- Bloods: ↑WCC, ↑ESR
- Cytogenetic analysis: t(11;22) translocation in tumour cells
- Radiograph:
  - Lytic lesions, soft tissue swelling, 'onion-skin' new bone
- MRI and bone biopsy (pustular appearance, small round blue cells)
- CT of the chest for metastases.

Management
- Neo-adjuvant and postoperative chemotherapy and excision +/– reconstruction:
  - Radiotherapy used for some cases
  - Amputation may be required
- Five-year survival of approximately 50–75% with modern treatments.

Chondrosarcoma

Chondrosarcoma is a rare malignant chondrogenic tumour of bone affecting older people (40–75 years) and mainly the metaphyses of long bones, pelvis, shoulder girdle and spine. Histological grades I–III are seen.

Presentation

- Bone pain and swelling
- Pathological fracture
- Spinal cord compression.

Investigations

- Radiograph:
  - Lytic/blastic lesions, soft tissue swelling, cortical destruction and 'popcorn' appearance
- MRI and bone biopsy
- CT for staging.

Management

- Surgical resection is the mainstay of management
- No response to chemotherapy or radiotherapy
- Five-year survival is dependent on grade.

Secondary Bone Tumours

Bone is the third most commonly affected site for metastases after the lung and liver. Secondary bone tumours often metastasize from the prostate, breast, kidney, lung, thyroid or skin. Haematogenous is the normal mode of spread.

Presentation

- Symptoms from primary lesion, e.g. haemoptysis and shortness of breath in lung cancer
- Systemic symptoms, e.g. malaise and weight loss
- Metabolic upset, e.g. hypercalcaemia leading to muscle weakness, polyuria and confusion
- Bone pain or pathological fracture:
  - Risk assessment done using the Mirel's scoring system
- Spinal cord compression (thoracic spine is a common site of metastases).

Investigations

- Bloods (elevated serum calcium, phosphate and ALP)
- Radiographs of affected region
- CT/MRI +/− bone biopsy:
  - Determine primary if not already known.

Management

- Analgesia, bisphosphonates and steroids for cord compression
- Radiotherapy and chemotherapy guided by primary malignancy
- Surgery:
  - Cord decompression
  - Stabilize actual or impending pathological fracture.

 HINTS AND TIPS

SECONDARY BONE TUMOURS

Older patients can present acutely with a pathological fracture through a lytic lesion in the bone. It is wrong to presume this a secondary bone tumour and to proceed with intramedullary nailing. Routine investigations and workup, including a biopsy, are required to determine the site of the primary malignancy or whether the lesion is a primary bone tumour.

NERVE INJURIES

 OVERVIEW

Clinical assessment with neurophysiological studies will often provide a definitive diagnosis for injuries or compression of a nerve. Management is dependent on the grade of nerve damage and the associated disability. This includes splints, physiotherapy, steroid injection, nerve decompression, nerve graft and tendon transfers.

Grades of Nerve Injury

Nerve injuries are commonly classified according to the Seddon classification:

- Neurapraxia (local demyelination; recovery 1–3 weeks)
- Axonotmesis (nerve axon death, nerve tube intact; recovery 1–3 mm/24 hours)
- Neurotmesis (nerve axon death, nerve tube transected or crushed; recovery 1–3 mm/24 hours but incomplete even with surgery).

Presentations of Nerve Injury

See Table 6.8 for the causes and presentations of nerve injuries to the lower limb, and injuries to the upper limb are discussed next. See Chapter 4 for some of the nerve injuries associated with common trauma.

TABLE 6.8
CAUSES AND PRESENTATION OF LOWER LIMB NERVE INJURIES

The tibial and common peroneal nerves are susceptible to external pressures, e.g. tight casts

Nerve	Cause(s)	Presentation
Sciatic	Pelvic fracture Posterior hip dislocation Iatrogenic	Sensory loss below knee (saphenous nerve spared) Motor loss of hamstrings and muscles below knee
Tibial	Tibial fracture Compartment syndrome Iatrogenic	Sensory loss over the sole of the foot Foot plantar and toe flexion loss Muscle wasting in sole of foot (chronic) Toe clawing
Common peroneal	Proximal fibula fracture Compartment syndrome Ganglion Iatrogenic	Foot drop (loss of dorsiflexion from deep peroneal nerve and eversion from superficial) High-stepping gait Sensory loss of dorsum foot and lower lateral aspect of leg

Brachial Plexus

Injury to the brachial plexus commonly follows a traction injury that forces the shoulder and neck apart, or one that pulls the arm upwards. Both types of injury are possible with complicated vaginal deliveries, e.g. breech birth. High-energy trauma (may damage an entire brachial plexus) or severely displaced pectoral girdle fractures are more common precipitants in adults. Radiographs (C-spine and CXR) with MRI of the C-spine may aid with determining the cause. Potential presentations are (please see Chapter 1):

- C5-C6 roots affected (Erb paralysis):
  - Arm adducted, forearm pronated, and palm upwards and backwards (waiter's tip position)
- C8-T1 roots affected (Klumpke's palsy):
  - Claw hand as intrinsic muscles of hand affected
  - Sensory loss in dermatome distribution
  - Associated with Horner's syndrome, Pancoast tumour and a cervical rib.

Axillary Nerve

Injury to the axillary nerve most commonly occurs following an anterior shoulder dislocation or a proximal humeral fracture (when the axillary nerve passes around the surgical neck of the humerus). Presentation is with paraesthesia or sensory loss over the lateral aspect of the upper arm ('regimental badge sign'), with shoulder abduction predominantly lost due to paralysis of the deltoid muscle.

Radial Nerve

Injury or compression of the radial nerve most commonly occurs as it passes around the spinal groove of the humerus. A neurapraxia can occur due to compression in the axilla either due to axillary crutches or when an intoxicated person passes out with an arm draping over a chair – 'Saturday night palsy'.

Isolated posterior interosseous nerve injury or compression may occur as the nerve passes between the two heads of the supinator and then circumnavigates the radial neck. This can be associated with repetitive trauma, e.g. pronation–supination movement, or trauma/iatrogenic injury (postsurgery) following a fracture and/or dislocation of the proximal radius.

PRESENTATIONS

- Paralysis of the wrist, thumb and finger extensors, leading to wrist drop and decreased grip strength:
  - A higher lesion will affect elbow extension also
- Forearm or triceps muscle wasting possible
- Sensory loss of a small area of the dorsum of the hand, i.e. first web space:
  - Posterior forearm if a higher lesion
- Posterior interosseous nerve injury alone will preserve elbow extension, and some wrist extension through extensor carpi radialis longus.

Ulnar Nerve

Injury or compression of the ulnar nerve most commonly occurs as it passes through the arcade of Struthers, posteriorly around the medial condyle of the elbow and through the cubital tunnel, or as it travels adjacent to the hook of hamate in the wrist in Guyon canal. Cubital tunnel syndrome is the second most common compressive neuropathy after carpal tunnel syndrome.

Precipitating factors for compression or injury include pregnancy, RA or OA leading to bony deformity at the elbow, e.g. cubitus valgus, myxoedema, elbow or hook of hamate fracture, elbow dislocation, repeated pressure at the elbow or wrist, or ganglion. AP and lateral radiographs of the elbow will help any potential bony pathology.

- Pain and paraesthesia of the medial side of the elbow with radiation to the ulnar distribution (sensory loss in little finger and ulnar half of ring finger).
- Hand intrinsic muscle (hypothenar, 3rd and 4th lumbricals, adductor pollicis and interossei) weakness and wasting with paralysis and potentially hand clawing:
  - Ulnar paradox: compression of the ulnar nerve at elbow results in less severe clawing due to weakness of FDP of medial two digits.
- Tardy ulnar nerve palsy: slow onset post-injury (years) that is often associated with cubitus valgus.

Median Nerve

Injury or compression (see carpal tunnel syndrome in this chapter) of the median nerve can occur. With trauma it is most common following an elbow, forearm (anterior interosseous nerve) or wrist fracture/laceration. Compression of the nerve at the elbow can occur between the heads of pronator teres (pronator syndrome).

PRESENTATIONS

- High lesion/injury, e.g. at the elbow:
  - Paralysis of pronation, wrist palmar flexion, thumb IPJ flexion
  - Muscle wasting of the forearm flexor compartment (anterior interosseous nerve)
  - Sensory loss of the lateral palm (preserved in carpal tunnel syndrome) and radial 3.5 digits.
- Low lesion/injury, e.g. at the wrist (see carpal tunnel syndrome):
  - Thenar muscle and radial two lumbrical paralysis +/– atrophy
  - Sensory loss of the radial 3.5 digits.

Chapter 7

Paediatric Orthopaedics and Rheumatology

BONE STRUCTURE AND INJURY

Structure of Young Bone

A normal long bone consists of the metaphysis, diaphysis and epiphysis. In growing bone, the epiphyseal plates have not fused (Figure 7.1) and thus injury to these parts of growing bone can cause growth disturbance leading to complications in later life, such as shortening and angular deformity. However, if the growth plate is not damaged some initial deformity after fracture healing may remodel to normality. In addition, children's bones heal more rapidly than those of adults.

Fracture Types in Children

The fracture classification system laid out in Chapter 4 can also be used for children. However, due to the bone being more elastic some fracture types only occur in children. These include:

- Greenstick fracture (Figure 7.2): a fracture where the bone bends as it does not fracture completely across, i.e. one side of the cortex often remains intact. Angulation and instability of the fracture are possible.
- Buckle fracture (Figure 7.3): a fracture where the bone buckles but no fracture line is seen, i.e. the cortex often remains intact. Angulation and instability of the fracture are uncommon.

Growth Plate Fracture

Five patterns of injury involving the growth plate in children are described in the Salter–Harris classification (Figure 7.4):

1. A transverse fracture with complete displacement along the epiphyseal plate line only.
2. Epiphysis detachment due to fracture, with an attached metaphysis fragment. This is the commonest type of fracture.
3. A displaced epiphyseal fracture fragment.

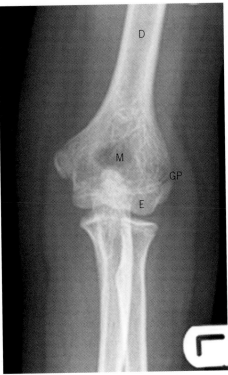

FIGURE 7.1

The anatomy of growing bone. The ossification of growth plates at the elbow are of particular importance. In ascending order of age of visualization (**CRITOL**): **c**apitellum (1 year old), **r**adial head (3 years old), **i**nternal/medial epicondyle (6 years old), **t**rochlea (8 years old), **o**lecranon (10 years old), and **l**ateral epicondyle (12 years old). D, diaphysis; E, epiphysis; GP, growth plate; M, metaphysis.

4. A fracture line that propagates through the epiphysis, epiphyseal plate and metaphysis.
5. Compression injury leading to obliteration of the epiphyseal growth plate.

A sixth pattern of fracture has been described, since production of the original classification, by Peterson. This is a severe injury of a localized section of the epiphysis, epiphyseal plate and metaphysis due to crush or burn (Figure 7.4). In types 3–6 the epiphyseal plate is very susceptible to growth disturbance due to premature growth plate fusion.

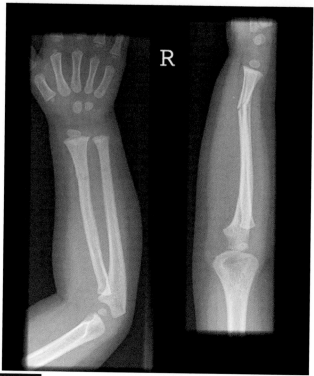

FIGURE 7.2

Greenstick diaphyseal fractures of the distal third of the radius and ulna.

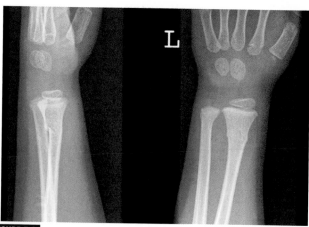

FIGURE 7.3

Buckle fracture of the distal radius.

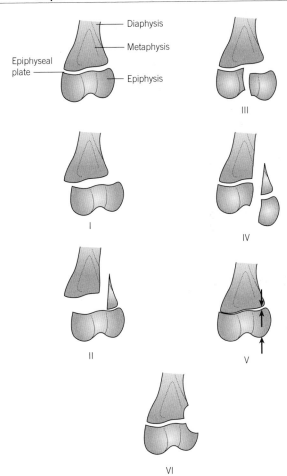

Salter–Harris classification of injury that involves the epiphyseal plate. Fractures commonly occur in the hypertrophic region of the plate. Peterson classification adds a type VI fracture to the original Salter–Harris classification.

HINTS AND TIPS

BONE STRUCTURE AND INJURY

Bone in childhood is more elastic than in adulthood. Salter–Harris classification is useful for guiding treatment as well as prognosticating the risk for growth problems following injury.

INJURIES IN CHILDREN

 OVERVIEW

As in adults, any bone may be fractured in children. The principles of treatment depend on degree of displacement, remodelling potential, fracture stability, growth-plate or joint-surface involvement as well as the requirement for pain relief. Always be aware of nonaccidental injury in children.

Humeral Supracondylar Fractures

Supracondylar fractures are most common in children aged 3–10 years old following a fall onto an extended (outstretched) hand. Posterior (extension type) displacement of the distal fragment is most commonly seen.

Presentation

Elbow pain, tenderness, swelling and possible deformity. It is essential to assess the neurovascular status of the affected limb (radial and brachial pulse, capillary refill time, median/anterior interosseous, ulnar and radial nerves – Chapters 1 and 2). An anterior interosseous nerve palsy is most commonly seen.

Investigations

- AP and lateral X-rays of the injured elbow (Figure 7.5):
  - Degree and direction of displacement determined:
    - Gartland classification (type 1: none; type 2: displacement with intact posterior cortex; type 3: completely displaced)
  - Radiocapitellar and anterior humeral line (Figure 7.6)
  - Baumann angle:
    - AP view of the elbow
    - The angle subtended by a line through the growth plate of the capitellum or lateral condylar physis with a line through the long axis of the humerus (normal ~70–75°).

Management

Dependent on the degree of displacement, with the timing dependent on the clinical presentation, in particular the presence of a vascular injury that is a surgical emergency.

- Fractures with no or minimal displacement (type 1 and some type 2) can be treated with immobilization in an above-elbow cast (elbow at 90°) for approximately 3-4 weeks, if there is no evidence of rotational deformity.
- Fractures with displacement (type 2 and type 3) can be treated with closed (open if not attainable) reduction under general anaesthesia, followed by fixation with K-wires.

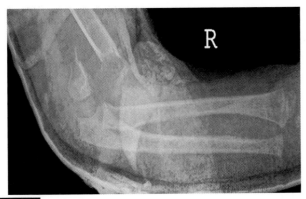

FIGURE 7.5

Grossly displaced supracondylar fracture of the humerus.

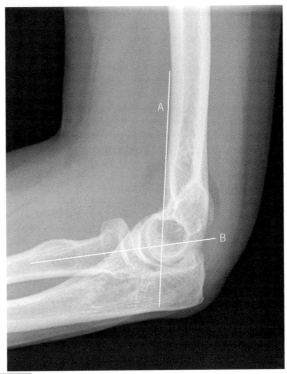

FIGURE 7.6

An elevated posterior fat pad may be a useful sign indicative of occult elbow pathology when no overt fracture is seen. The anterior humeral line should intersect the anterior half of the capitellum (**A**). A displaced radiocapitellar line is indicative of an elbow or radial head dislocation (**B**).

- It is essential to determine the neurovascular status of the affected limb both before and after reduction, as well as performing a postreduction radiograph.

Complications

These include stiffness, infection, malunion, compartment syndrome, neurovascular injury (brachial artery and major nerves including AIN), heterotopic ossification (stiffness) and long-term deformity (e.g. cubitus varus – known as a 'gun-stock' deformity).

Fractures of the Humeral Condyles

Medial epicondyle (9–14 years) fractures are relatively uncommon in children, with lateral condyle (5–10 years) fractures more frequently seen.

Presentation

Elbow pain, tenderness and swelling, with lateralization to the affected side. It is essential to determine the neurovascular status of the affected limb (radial and brachial pulse, capillary refill time, ulnar nerve).

Investigations

- AP and lateral views of the injured elbow:
  - May only show an elevated posterior fat pad (Figure 7.6)
  - Medial epicondyle fractures are associated with a dislocation of the elbow in ~50% of cases and require reduction in the emergency department
  - Lateral condyle fractures:
    - Salter–Harris IV pattern is common (Milch classification)
    - Internal oblique view to define displacement.

Management

Dependent on the degree of displacement and the side affected:

- Medial epicondyle fractures are routinely managed nonoperatively, even when displaced:
  - Absolute indication for surgery includes incarceration of fragment in joint, severe displacement and ulnar nerve injury.
- Lateral condyle injuries: fractures with minimal displacement (<2 mm) can be treated with immobilization in an above-elbow cast, but must be monitored closely for displacement. Fractures with displacement can be treated with reduction (routinely open) and fixation (K-wire or screws).

Complications

These include AVN, malunion or nonunion (leading to cubitus valgus), neurovascular injury (e.g. tardy ulnar nerve palsy), recurrent dislocation, growth arrest and long-term deformity.

Pulled Elbow

A pulled elbow is common following a 'yank' on a toddler's wrist leading to subluxation of the radial head out of the annular ligament. Clinical presentation is with elbow pain on forced extension. Investigations are only required when the diagnosis is in doubt. Management is by immediate gentle reduction routinely using supination and elbow flexion.

Forearm Fractures

Forearm fractures are the most common site of injury in children. Injury most commonly occurs following a fall onto an extended (outstretched) hand. Both bone fractures commonly follow a higher energy injury, e.g. fall from a height. Types of fracture include:

- Diaphyseal fractures (single or both bone):
  - Greenstick fractures
  - Complete
- Distal physeal and metaphyseal fractures:
  - Growth plate fractures, most commonly Salter–Harris type 2
  - Buckle fractures
- Fracture + dislocation:
  - Monteggia or Galeazzi fractures (see Chapter 6).

Presentation

Forearm and/or wrist pain, tenderness and swelling, with dorsal displacement of the distal fragment(s) are common. Gross deformity may be apparent. It is again essential to determine the neurovascular status of the affected limb and if there is an open injury, which can be subtle, e.g. puncture wound.

Investigations

AP and lateral views of the injured wrist/forearm/elbow (Figure 7.7).

Management

This is dependent on the type and location of the fracture, as well as the age of the patient and the degree of displacement (Table 7.1). Reduction is routinely via MUA, with immobilization in an above-elbow POP with moulding. Supplementary K-wire fixation for fractures of the distal radius can

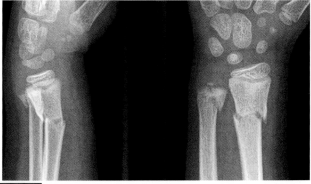

FIGURE 7.7

A distal radial fracture with ~30° dorsal angulation. There is a Salter–Harris type 4 fracture of the distal ulna.

TABLE 7.1	
TREATMENT OPTIONS FOR FOREARM FRACTURES IN CHILDREN	
Fracture type	**Treatment options***
Buckle	Immobilization with splint or plaster
Greenstick:	
<15–20° angulation	Immobilization with plaster
>15–20° angulation	Reduction followed by immobilization with plaster (X-ray check at 1 week)
Growth plate or complete fractures:†	
Stable postreduction	Reduction followed by immobilization with plaster (X-ray check at 1 week)
Unstable postreduction	Consider internal fixation, e.g. with K-wires or nailing

*Other factors, including remodelling potential and age, need to be considered when determining optimal treatment. The degree of deformity is not the only factor.
†Salter–Harris type 3 and 4 fractures require an anatomical reduction.

be required if instability is present. For forearm fractures, elastic nailing or ORIF can be used when indicated.

Complications

Uncommon but include malunion, nonunion, compartment syndrome and re-fracture.

Femoral Shaft Fractures

Femoral shaft fractures are most frequently seen in toddlers (2–4 years of age) and in adolescents, with falls and higher energy injuries the common respective mechanisms of injury. Nonaccidental injury must always be considered, particularly in the pre-walking child.

Presentation

Thigh pain, tenderness, swelling and possibly deformity present with an inability to mobilize. It is essential to assess the neurovascular status of the affected limb.

Investigations

- AP and lateral X-rays of the femur:
  - Degree and direction of displacement
  - Ensure adequate views of hip and knee are obtained.

Management

Dependent on the age, weight and degree of displacement:

- Babies and infants (<18 months): gallows/hoop traction +/– hip spica
- Toddlers (18 months – 4 years): traction (e.g. Thomas splint, Hamilton–Russell) +/– hip spica
- Children (4–12 years): intramedullary elastic nailing or ORIF.

Complications

These include leg length discrepancy, malunion, nonunion, re-fracture and AVN of the femoral head.

Tibial Fractures

Tibial fractures are a common lower limb injury in children and are commonly divided into:

- Diaphyseal:
    - Toddler's fracture (low energy rotational injury)
    - Tibial shaft +/− fibula (higher energy)
- Distal tibial:
    - Tillaux fracture (Salter–Harris type 3 fracture of anterolateral distal tibia epiphysis)
    - Triplane fracture (Salter–Harris type 4):
        - Fracture in three planes: Epiphysis-sagittal, metaphysic-coronal and physis-axial.
        - Appears to be Salter-Harris 3 on the AP and Salter-Harris 2 on the lateral radiographs.

Presentation

Leg/ankle pain, tenderness, swelling and possibly deformity present with an inability to mobilize and reduced range of movement at the ankle and knee. It is essential to assess the neurovascular status of the affected limb, for any open injuries and for any clinical evidence of compartment syndrome (see Chapter 4).

Investigations

- AP and lateral X-rays of the tibia and fibula:
    - Degree and direction of displacement
    - Ensure adequate views of ankle and knee are obtained
- CT scan:
    - Often required to further delineate fractures of the distal tibia, particularly for the triplane fracture.

Management

It is dependent on the age, fracture type and degree of displacement. Options include:

- Nonoperative:
    - Long-leg casting with moulding +/− closed reduction for undisplaced and minimally displaced fractures and toddler's fractures
- Operative:
    - Plate fixation or intramedullary elastic nailing for diaphyseal fractures.
    - ORIF for displaced distal tibial fractures (occasionally closed reduction is possible)

Complications

These include residual pain and stiffness, compartment syndrome, diaphyseal malunion (varus for isolated tibial fractures, valgus for tibia and fibula fractures), nonunion and early growth arrest for physeal injuries.

HINTS AND TIPS

INJURIES IN CHILDREN

It is essential to be vigilant for nonaccidental injury in children, as almost two-thirds of children who die as a consequence of abuse will have had prior consultations with healthcare and/or social services. Aspects that may suggest nonaccidential injury include a delay in presentation, a changing history of the injury or one that is not consistent with the age of the child or the injury sustained (e.g. a femoral fracture in a nonambulator), abnormal interaction and behaviour of carers with physician and/or child, and several fractures/injuries of varying duration. A full assessment is essential and referral to the child protection team.

DISORDERS OF THE HIP

 OVERVIEW

The limping child is a common presentation to both primary and secondary care. Although definable pathology is not identified in the majority of cases, a thorough clinical assessment and investigation is required to rule out common causes. The differential diagnosis of a childhood limp is found in Table 7.2.

Developmental Dysplasia of the Hip

This congenital abnormality is relatively common. At birth the incidence of hip instability is 5–20/1000, whilst at 3 weeks this proportion has dropped to 1.5/1000 due to natural stabilization of the hip joint during this period. The left hip is more commonly affected (4:1) but it occurs bilaterally in 10–30% of cases.

Pathogenesis

The preterm acetabulum is naturally shallow with a sloping roof. DDH occurs where the femoral head does not sit centrally within its socket causing the joint capsule to be stretched. The femoral head is displaced superiorly and

TABLE 7.2

THE IMPORTANT DIAGNOSES FOR A CHILD PRESENTING WITH A LIMP, CATEGORIZED BY SITE AND AGE

Site	Diagnosis	Usual Age Range
General	Osteomyelitis Septic arthritis Trauma Tumour	Any
Spine	Discitis	3 months to 8 years
Hip	DDH Perthes disease Transient synovitis Slipped upper femoral epiphysis	Infancy, but may be delayed 4–8 years 4–8 years 10–14 years

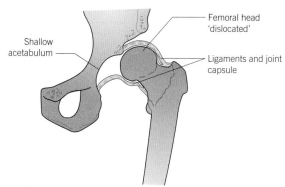

Femoral head 'dislocated'

Shallow acetabulum

Ligaments and joint capsule

FIGURE 7.8

Diagram showing the abnormal position of the femoral head relative to a shallow acetabulum (compare with Figure 7.10).

posteriorly (Figure 7.8), leading to impeded development of both the shallow acetabulum and proximal femur (head and neck). DDH includes a spectrum of abnormalities in the neonate:

- Shallow acetabulum with dysplasia (hip in joint and not dislocatable)
- Shallow acetabulum with dysplasia (hip in joint but dislocatable)
- Neonatal dislocation (reducible)
- Neonatal dislocation (irreducible; possibly because labrum, lax joint capsule and/or interposed soft tissues are within the joint)
- Frank subluxation/dislocation in an older child.

Risk Factors

- Genetic:
  - Increased probability in girls and if a relative has DDH, i.e. a family history of DDH
- Concomitant congenital deformities, e.g. plagiocephaly, torticollis, club foot, spinal deformity (neural tube defects), scoliosis, Down syndrome and metatarsus adductus
- Perinatal:
  - Prematurity
  - First born
  - Breech birth (1 in 5), large babies, oligohydramnios, multiple births, e.g. twins, premature, caesarian-section, first born
  - Poor postnatal care
  - Older mothers
  - Seen in certain populations, e.g. Inuit/Eskimos of North America.

Presentation (Early)

Examination of all babies for hip instability should occur at birth and at 6 weeks. Two tests that are commonly performed are described below:

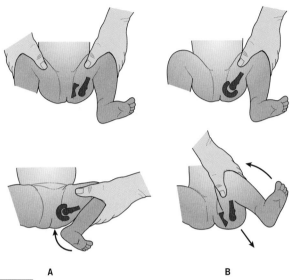

FIGURE 7.9
(**A**) Ortolani test. (**B**) Barlow test.

- Ortolani test (Figure 7.9A):
  - Supine, hips and knees bilaterally flexed to 90°
  - Place fingers over greater trochanters, with thumbs over inner thigh
  - Gently abduct both hips
  - Negative (normal) = complete and unimpeded 90° of hip abduction
  - Positive (DDH) = impeded abduction with a palpable and audible jerk as the femoral head reduces and enters the acetabulum, followed by full unimpeded hip abduction. If 90° abduction impossible the dislocation may be irreducible
- Barlow test (Figure 7.9B):
  - Supine, hips flexed to 90° and adducted
  - Stabilize pelvis with thumbs in the groin
  - Gently push the thighs posteriorly towards the couch
  - Negative (normal) = no dislocation of femoral head achieved
  - Positive (DDH) = femoral head slips over the posterior lip and out of the acetabulum and back in again, i.e. the hip is unstable and dislocating.

Presentation (Late)

Examination of babies at 6-month intervals during the first 2 years of life may identify late signs:

- Unilateral DDH:
  - Limited abduction of affected hip
  - Asymmetrical skin contours over thigh

- Delayed walking
- Trendelenburg gait due to a dysplastic hip giving a shortened leg with external rotation of the leg
- Bilateral DDH:
  - Fewer features
  - Impeded abduction at both hip joints
  - Broadened perineal space.

Investigations

- Ultrasound:
  - Early investigation (<25 weeks of age)
  - Determines the characteristics of the acetabulum, as well as the relative location of the femoral head
  - Potential screening tool
- Hip (AP and lateral) and pelvic radiographs:
  - Late investigation:
    - Femoral head and acetabulum are not clearly seen at birth. The femoral head should begin to ossify after 3 months of age.
  - May show a shallow acetabulum with a dislocated and immature femoral head
  - Shenton arc, Hilgenreiner and Perkin lines (Figure 7.10):
    - The femoral head ossification should be in the medial inferior quadrant of bisecting Hilgenreiner and Perkin lines.

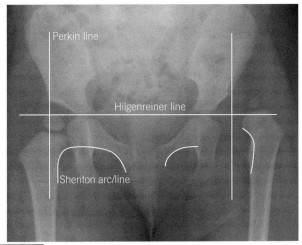

FIGURE 7.10

An AP pelvic radiograph demonstrating Shenton, Hilgenreiner and Perkin lines. Shenton line should be a continuous arc from the inferior border of femoral neck to the superior margin of the obturator foramen. Hilgenreiner line is a horizontal line that bisects the left and right triradiate cartilage. Perkin line runs perpendicular to Hilgenreiner line at the lateral edge of the acetabulum.

TABLE 7.3	

TREATMENT OPTIONS AT THE VARIOUS STAGES OF DDH*

Timing	Treatment Options
Early (<6 months)	Multiple nappies and reassessment with ultrasound within 3–6 weeks
	Moderate abduction splint with the hips flexed at 100°, e.g. Pavlik harness
Delayed (<6 years)	Gradual persistent traction then closed reduction and splintage
	Gradual persistent traction then open reduction ± femoral or pelvic osteotomy
Late (>6 years)	Open reduction ± femoral or pelvic osteotomy
	None (especially bilateral disorder)
	Delayed hip arthroplasty when highly symptomatic

*Since the hip is a deep-seated joint, imaging (ultrasound, radiograph, arthrogram) is required at all stages of treatment to confirm reduction and acetabular development.

Management

Diagnosis and treatment at birth give the best prognosis, with follow-up surveillance necessary for all confirmed, treated or at-risk cases. Treatment options depend on the timing and severity of presentation (Table 7.3). They include:

- Immobilization with an abduction splint:
  - Confirm reduction of femoral head and development of acetabulum using ultrasound
  - Pavlik harness or von Rosen splint
  - Avoid position of extreme abduction as there is a risk of avascular necrosis of the femoral head (Figure 7.11)
- Closed reduction
- Open reduction ± femoral varus derotation or pelvic osteotomy

Complications

The complications of frank dislocation are poor development of the acetabulum and femoral epiphysis, with subsequent secondary osteoarthritis. Osteonecrosis may be a complication of treatment.

Perthes Disease

Legg–Calvé–Perthes disease is an idiopathic osteonecrosis of the capital femoral epiphysis (femoral head). The incidence is ~1 in 12 000 and peaks between the ages of 4 and 8 years, but is seen between 3 and 11 years of age. It is more common in boys (4 : 1) and occurs bilaterally in 10–20% of cases. A better prognosis is seen with younger patients.

Pathogenesis

The cause of osteonecrosis in Perthes is uncertain. Ischaemic episodes may be due to one of several varied aetiologies including microemboli and retinacular vessel tamponade, which result in partial necrosis of the femoral head. The speed of the subsequent revascularization and healing of the necrotic zone, along with the extent of epiphyseal damage, determines whether the reossification and remodelling process that eventually occurs produces a

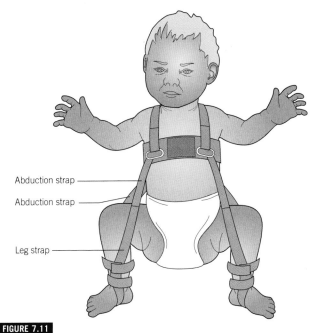

Abduction strap

Abduction strap

Leg strap

FIGURE 7.11

Pavlik harness used in the early treatment of DDH.

deformed femoral head that will cause joint incongruity (ball and socket do not match).

Risk Factors

- Genetic, e.g. family history of Perthes
- Perinatal (low birth weight)
- Socioeconomic (deprivation and secondhand smoking).

Presentation

- Hip and/or knee pain with an associated limp.
- Hip movements normal apart from reduced abduction and internal rotation.

Investigations

Four classification systems, based on radiological appearance, are commonly used to grade disease severity or determine outcome. They are:

- Catterall: proportion of femoral head affected, four grades
- Salter–Thompson: length of subchondral fracture line, two grades
- Herring (Figure 7.12): loss of lateral femoral head height, three grades
- Stulberg: congruency of hip joint.

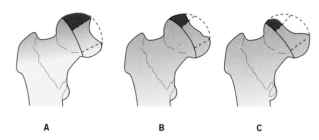

A Grade A: normal pillar height
B Grade B: >50% height maintained
C Grade C: <50% height maintained

FIGURE 7.12

The Herring (lateral pillar) classification is one of the most effective grading systems for the assessment of prognosis and treatment in Perthes disease.

The recommended investigations are:

- Hip (AP and lateral) and pelvic radiographs (Figure 7.13):
  - Early changes: ↑articular space; ↑density and ↓size of femoral head epiphysis; crescent sign (subchondral fracture line)
  - Late changes: fragmentation, fissuring, displacement, collapse and/or fracture of the femoral head epiphysis with subsequent deformity and remodelling; joint subluxation; lateral para-physeal rarefaction (Gage sign)
- MRI may confirm extent of osteonecrosis.

Management

Treatment options depend on the age of the child and the extent of osteonecrosis. The prognosis is better with a younger age of onset due to the increased remodelling potential:

- Mild to moderate disease:
  - Reduced activity until pain free
  - Physiotherapy
  - Follow-up with imaging is essential
- Moderate to severe disease:
  - Consider surgery with osteotomy of the femur and/or pelvis
  - Children >8 yrs (bone age >6 yrs), lateral pillar B and B/C stages are included in this group
- Severe disease: with a very deformed femoral head and acetabulum which are incongruent, the prognosis is poor and total hip replacement may be necessary in adulthood.

Complications

- Pain and loss of function
- Deformities, e.g. limb shortening and rotational deformity (severe joint incongruity is a cause of early-onset osteoarthritis)

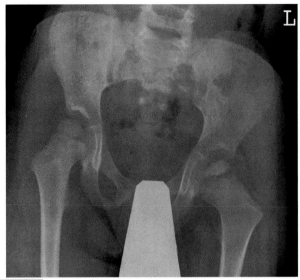

FIGURE 7.13

Perthes disease of the left hip. The left femoral epiphysis is flattened, irregular and mildly sclerotic. Metaphyseal and epiphyseal rarefaction are severe signs.

- Osteochondritis dissecans (separation of a necrotic fragment within the joint).

Slipped Upper Femoral Epiphysis

The overall incidence is ~5 per 100 000 population and peaks in pubescence (10–14 years of age). It is more common in boys (3:1) and occurs bilaterally in ~17–50% of cases, of which ~25% occur at the same time.

Pathogenesis

Slipped upper femoral epiphysis is characterized by a posterior–inferior displacement of the upper femoral epiphysis due to a stress fracture at the growth plate (a form of pathological Salter–Harris type 1 growth plate fracture). This is possibly due to a defect within the hyaline cartilage of the growth plate, or from excess force across it, e.g. in an overweight child. Potential associations include:

- Obesity (~60%)
- Endocrine disorders, e.g. hypothyroidism, growth hormone
- Renal failure
- History of radiotherapy (local/pituitary)
- Delayed onset puberty.

Presentation

- History of injury in about one-third of presentations:
  - Acute, chronic (<3 weeks) and acute on chronic
- Pain (groin, hip and/or knee)
- Limp (Loder classification):
  - Stable: able to weight bear with or without crutches – risk of AVN <10%
  - Unstable: unable to weight bear even with crutches – risk of AVN ~50%
- Decreased range of movement, in particular flexion, abduction and internal rotation
- Limb may be shortened and lie in external rotation.

Investigations

- Hip (AP and frog lateral) and pelvic radiographs (Figure 7.14):
  - Displacement of the head and severity of the slip can be measured by the percentage of the slip (0–33% mild, 34–50% moderate, >50% severe).
  - Trethowan sign is present if the continuation of a line (Klein's line) along the lateral edge of the femoral neck on the AP radiograph does not include any portion of the upper femoral epiphysis.

Management

No forced attempt is made to reduce the slip as this has a high risk of damaging the vascular supply to the femoral head leading to osteonecrosis:

- Mild displacement:
  - Screw fixation 'in-situ'

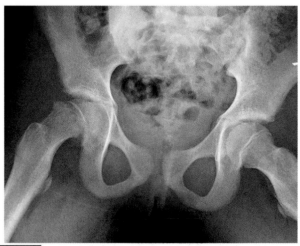

FIGURE 7.14

A slipped upper femoral epiphysis of the right hip. A SUFE is best seen on a 'frog-lateral' radiograph of the hips.

- Moderate displacement:
  - Screw fixation 'in-situ'
  - Consider femoral neck osteotomy for deformity
- Severe displacement:
  - Consider primary femoral neck osteotomy.

Complications

- Contralateral slip (prophylactic fixation advocated by some)
- Avascular necrosis of the femoral head, particularly if reduction is attempted
- Cam hip morphology after a mild slip causing femoro-acetabular impingement.
- Secondary arthritis due to coxa-vara (femoral head in varus) or avascular necrosis

Transient Synovitis of the Hip

Otherwise known as irritable hip, transient synovitis of the hip is a self-limiting inflammatory disorder of the hip joint. No cause has been identified as definitive. However, the following are thought to be related:

- History of injury
- Recent viral infection, e.g. respiratory tract
- Allergy.

The disorder is very common and peaks in prepubescence (3–10 years of age). It is more common in boys (2:1).

Presentation

- History of earlier viral infection of upper respiratory or gastro-intestinal tracts, or injury in some cases
- Pain (groin, hip and/or knee)
- Limp
- Decreased range of movement (mild)
- Involuntary muscle spasm
- Systemic upset, e.g. fever:
  - Always consider septic arthritis/osteomyelitis.

Investigations

- Blood tests:
  - Mildly raised ESR and WCC. If these markers, as well as CRP, are significantly raised, a diagnosis of sepsis must be considered
- Hip (AP and lateral) and pelvic radiographs:
  - Often normal and not routine in some centres
  - Exclude other causes
- Ultrasound:
  - Assess for effusion
- Joint aspiration as indicated (uncommon)
  - It is important to exclude septic arthritis so samples should be sent to for Gram stain and culture.

Management

- Bed rest for symptoms
- Nonsteroidal antiinflammatory analgesics (NSAIDs)
- Advise should improve within 2–3 weeks.

 HINTS AND TIPS

DISORDERS OF THE HIP

Knee pain along with a limp is a common presentation for hip pathology in children. The age of onset and history of presentation are key aids in the diagnosis of the common hip disorders in children. An in-toeing gait is a common reason for referral to the paediatric orthopaedic clinic. Common causes include persistent femoral neck anteversion, internal tibial torsion and metatarsus adductus, most of which correct as the child grows.

DISORDERS OF THE KNEE

Patellar instability is discussed in Chapter 6.

Osteochondritis Dissecans

Osteochondritis dissecans can occur at any joint, but is commonly seen in the knees. It is characterized by osteochondral fracture or separation of a region of the maturing epiphysis in susceptible children, especially the medial femoral condyle. The cause may be traumatic, although bilateral disease is not infrequent. In children, the fragment rarely detaches, and healing is the norm. Two other specific types of osteochondritis (traction apophysitis) found in the knee are:

- Osgood–Schlatter disease: tibial tuberosity
- Sinding–Larsen–Johansson syndrome: inferior pole of patella.

Presentation

- Pain in the knee:
  - May be localized to the affected bone, e.g. over the tibial tuberosity
  - Sporadic
  - Worse at maximal extension, internal rotation and flexion, but with full range of movement
- Swelling, effusion or locking of the joint
- Limp.

Investigations

- Knee (AP and lateral) radiographs:
  - Area of high density (sclerosis)
  - Osseous fragmentation
  - Loose body (rare)
- MRI to identify fragment stability.

Management

- Analgesia
- Physiotherapy, rest and/or immobilization

- Surgery (rare):
  - Pin fixation or removal of displaced bone fragment.

 HINTS AND TIPS

DISORDERS OF THE KNEE

It is important to remember that from birth children have bowlegs (genu varum). By 2–3 years old this has progressed to genu valgum (knock-knees). This then stabilizes at 7 years of age to approximately 7–9° of valgus. Pathological causes for a persistent deformity include trauma, skeletal dysplasias, benign tumours, Blount's disease (severe idiopathic tibia vara) and rickets. Unilateral deformity should be investigated.

DISORDERS OF THE FOOT

Club Foot (Congenital Talipes Equinovarus)

This disorder has an incidence of 1–4/1000 births, with a higher figure seen in the developing world. It is more common in boys (2–3 : 1), and occurs bilaterally in 30–50% of cases. Recurrence is common following treatment that requires intensive and long-term passive splinting.

Pathogenesis

Neonatal club foot is associated with atrophy and growth failure of the calf and medial soft tissues (e.g. joint capsule and tibialis posterior) leading to a characteristic deformity of the foot:

- Fixed equinus (foot is fixed in plantar flexion)
- Total hindfoot inversion with direction towards the midline (varus position)
- Adduction and supination of the midfoot and forefoot relative to the hindfoot.

Risk factors

- Genetic:
  - Increased probability if a relative is affected, i.e. a family history of club foot
  - Concomitant congenital deformities, e.g. DDH, spina bifida, myelomeningocoele, arthrogryposis and trisomy 21
- Perinatal:
  - Maternal alcohol, smoking and/or intravenous drug use.

Presentation

- May be identified at 20-week prenatal scan; however, 'false positives' are common and frequently resolve spontaneously during the third trimester
- Apparent at birth
- Decreased range of movement with passive foot eversion and dorsiflexion limited
- Calf muscle wasting
- Leg shortening due to shortening of the tibia.

TABLE 7.4

TREATMENT OPTIONS AT THE VARIOUS STAGES OF CONGENITAL TALIPES EQUINOVARUS

Timing	Treatment Options
Early	Ponseti method*
	Regular manipulations of the affected foot/feet
	Maintain repositioning with splint or plaster
Delayed	Ponseti method*
	Consider surgical release of the posterior compartment and lengthening of the muscles and tendons >9 months of age
	Maintain correction with fixation and splints
Late	Consider surgical release, removal of soft tissue and bone respectively
	Triple arthrodesis >8–10 years of age

*Ponseti method includes an Achilles tenotomy in 80% of cases.

Investigations

- Foot radiographs (bilateral AP and dorsiflexion lateral):
  - Altered position of the talus relative to the calcaneus (Kite angle)
  - Subluxation of the talonavicular joint.

There are many classification systems that can be used to grade disease severity and/or determine treatment and outcome. Those commonly employed are Pirani, Harold–Walker, Goldner and Dimeglio classifications.

Management (Table 7.4)

Treatment options depend on the timing of presentation and response to treatment, but none is cosmetically definitive. They include:

- Conservative:
  - The Ponseti method is a popular modern method of treatment which is mainly nonoperative:
    - Employs a series of manoeuvres and sequential casting, followed by foot abduction orthoses up to the age of 5 yrs
    - Corrects deformity over time
    - Reported success rates ~90–95%
  - Physiotherapy
  - Immobilization in the correct position using plastering or strapping
- Surgical:
  - Posterior release with lengthening of the posterior and/or medial soft tissues followed by postoperative immobilization (e.g. Denis Browne splint)
  - Release and removal of soft tissue and bone, respectively
  - Triple arthrodesis (fusion of subtalar, talonavicular and calcaneocuboid joints) for delayed presentation or late recurrence.

Complications

If the abnormality is not corrected early enough, growth leads to permanent and abnormal secondary bone and joint changes. Post-treatment complications include:

- Pain, stiffness and muscle weakness
- Avascular necrosis of the talus
- Recurrence and/or deformity.

 HINTS AND TIPS

DISORDERS OF THE FOOT

Flat feet are common under 3 years of age until the development of the medial longitudinal arch. A persistent flexible flat foot, i.e. tiptoe stance restores arch and heel moves into varus, does not require investigation or treatment. A persistent rigid flat foot that does not correct on tiptoe stance can be associated tarsal coalition, congenital vertical talus or an undiagnosed inflammatory disorders and requires further investigation.

JUVENILE IDIOPATHIC ARTHRITIS

 OVERVIEW

Juvenile idiopathic arthritis (JIA) is defined as an inflammatory arthritis beginning before the age of 17 that persists for at least 6 weeks, where other causes such as infection have been excluded.

The estimated annual incidence in the UK is about 1 in 10 000. The term JIA is also used when the condition persists into adulthood since about 50% of children with JIA go into adult life with active disease. The disorder is more common in girls overall, but boys are more commonly affected in some disease subgroups.

Pathogenesis

The cause of JIA is unknown but like other autoimmune diseases, genetic and environmental factors are thought to be involved. There is a strong association with HLA variants but these differ from those involved in adult RA. Other variants close to or within cytokine genes and genes involved in regulating the immune response also play a role. As in adult forms of inflammatory arthritis, JIA is characterized by an inflammatory infiltrate of affected joints resulting in the production of proinflammatory cytokines, such as TNFα, IL-6 and IL-1, which promote destruction of bone, cartilage and soft tissues.

Presentation

The clinical presentation varies with subtype (Table 7.5). The arthritis presents with pain, morning stiffness and inactivity gelling. The presenting feature is often a limp if the lower limb joints are affected or a reluctance to use an arm for upper limb involvement. Uveitis is a common complication. In toddlers the presentation can be subtle and easily missed. Systemic JIA presents with a systemic illness accompanied by rash and fever. Joint pain and stiffness may also be present but the systemic features can occur before arthritis develops.

Extraarticular Features

- Uveitis:
  - Most common in oligoarticular disease but also occurs in early rheumatoid arthritis (ERA), juvenile PsA and undifferentiated forms of JIA

TABLE 7.5

JUVENILE IDIOPATHIC ARTHRITIS SUBTYPES AND PRESENTATIONS

Subtype	Presentation	Comment
Oligoarthritis (50%)	1–4 joints affected within 6 months Young girls (~3 years) Positive ANA and/or HLA-DR5 (50%)	Often complicated by uveitis. Prognosis good when few joints involved but poor with extending arthritis.
Persisting	Asymmetrical in the lower limbs (knees and ankles) No systemic disturbance and RF negative	
Extending	25–30% of these patients Progressive polyarthritis after 6 months	
Polyarthritis (35%) RF negative (90%)	5 or more joints affected within 6 months Young girls, symmetrical, any joint in all four limbs Cervical spine (results in surgical cervical fusion) TMJ (poorly matured mandible and receding chin)	Prognosis poor, often persists into adulthood
RF positive (10%)	Older girls (>8 years) Similar course to RA (e.g. hands and wrists) Erosions, joint destruction, nodules and systemic effects Association with HLA-DR4	
Systemic arthritis (10%)	Arthritis with fever for >2 weeks (Still disease) Young girls and boys Intermittent pyrexia (>2 weeks) with a maculopapular rash, arthritis, lymphadenopathy, myalgia, hepatosplenomegaly, pericarditis, anaemia and pleurisy Raised inflammatory markers and a thrombocytosis	Recurrence common. Complications include chronic polyarthritis and amyloidosis
Other (5%) Psoriatic arthritis	Arthritis (few joints but destructive) + psoriasis, or Arthritis + family history of psoriasis + nail pitting or dactylitis Form seen in children is similar to that found in adults	May be complicated by uveitis
Enthesitis arthritis	Older boys, asymmetrical in the lower limb Arthritis + enthesitis or arthritis + two of the associated features: sacroiliitis, HLA-B27 (75%), anterior uveitis and a family history of spondyloarthritis, uveitis or IBD	Progresses to ankylosing spondylitis in adulthood

TMJ, temporomandibular joint.

- Hepatosplenomegaly, lymphadenopathy and fever:
  - Key features of systemic JIA
- Rash:
  - Systemic JIA and juvenile PsA
- Pleural or pericardial effusions:
  - Systemic JIA
- Unequal limb length due to premature fusion of epiphysis:
  - All forms of inflammatory arthritis
- Amyloidosis
- Growth retardation (due to corticosteroid treatment)
- Osteoporosis.

Investigations

- Routine bloods: normochromic normocytic anaemia, thrombocytosis, raised ESR and CRP (especially systemic JIA and polyarticular JIA)
- Immunology: CCP and RF negative (except in RA-like subtype); ANA usually positive in oligoarticular and polyarticular JIA
- Synovial fluid: sterile, and cloudy with raised WCC and low viscosity
- Imaging: erosions on X-ray with advanced disease in affected synovial joints; fusion of epiphysis of affected joints; and sacroiliitis on MRI in early rheumatoid arthritis subtype.

Management

OLIGOARTICULAR DISEASE

Therapy with NSAIDs is required in most cases for symptomatic relief, but this does not have a disease modifying effect. Intraarticular corticosteroids may be highly effective at inducing remission of arthritis for prolonged periods especially in oligoarticular disease. Methotrexate (15 mg/kg/m^2) is the second-line agent of choice in patients that do not respond adequately to NSAIDs and intraarticular corticosteroids. Sulfasalazine can be of value in oligoarticular disease but side effects are common and anti-TNF agents are often used for patients that do not respond to methotrexate. Abatacept may be successful in patients who fail to respond to TNFi therapy.

SYSTEMIC JUVENILE IDIOPATHIC ARTHRITIS

The first-line therapy is NSAIDs and intraarticular corticosteroids. Patients that did not respond adequately have traditionally been given systemic corticosteroids, but biologicals including anakinra, canakinumab and tocilizumab have all been found to be efficacious and are being used with increasing frequency.

UVEITIS

Referral to an ophthalmologist is advised. First-line therapy is with local corticosteroid drops and mydriatic eye drops. Patients who do not respond may require methotrexate and/or anti-TNF therapy.

NONPHARMACOLOGICAL APPROACHES

- Education and joint protection strategies
- Splints, appliances and household aids

- Rest during disease flares
- Physiotherapy to encourage joint movement and maintain muscle power.

SURGERY

Has an important role in patients with mechanical damage to joints or tendons or when response to optimal medical management is inadequate. Procedures include:

- Joint replacement surgery
- Tendon repair
- Synovectomy.

Prognosis

About 50% of patients go into remission but 50% have persistent inflammatory disease into adulthood. Poor prognostic features include:

- Polyarticular involvement
- Systemic involvement.

 HINTS AND TIPS

JUVENILE IDIOPATHIC ARTHRITIS

A multidisciplinary approach is essential in the management of JIA and should include physicians, surgeons, specialist nurses, physiotherapists, occupational therapists and clinical psychologists.

Chapter 8

Therapeutics

CHAPTER OUTLINE

PAIN MANAGEMENT
CORTICOSTEROIDS
DISEASE-MODIFYING
ANTIRHEUMATIC DRUGS
BIOLOGICAL ANTIRHEUMATIC
DRUGS

DRUGS FOR BONE DISEASES
HYPERURICAEMIA AND GOUT
ANTICOAGULANTS

We recommend that the first point of reference when prescribing is the BNF or an equivalent recognized drug formulary. Some of these medications will be used in community practice and in other specialties. The aim of this chapter is to provide more detailed information on the drugs commonly used within orthopaedics and rheumatology.

Most of the drug tables in this chapter were originally from the *In Clinical Practice Series: Arthritis*, Churchill Livingstone, 2004, Panayi and Dickson, ISBN 9780443074677. Updated by kind permission of Dr John Dickson.

PAIN MANAGEMENT

Management of pain is an essential part of any surgical or medical specialty. The World Health Organisation (WHO) pain ladder is found in Figure 8.1. Details of commonly used drugs for pain control are summarized in Tables 8.1–8.4.

Paracetamol

Paracetamol (also known as acetaminophen) is a widely used analgesic for mild to moderate pain and is the first choice analgesic in osteoarthritis. Paracetamol can be used alone or in combination with NSAIDs, opioids or other analgesics.

Opioids

Opioids are a class of powerful analgesics that act on both the central and peripheral nervous systems. The analgesic effects of opioids are thought to be mainly mediated by binding to the μ-class of opioid receptors, although there are two other receptor subtypes (κ and δ). Opioids have a number of unwanted effects also mediated by the same pathways including constipation, nausea, vomiting, somnolence, itching, dizziness and respiratory depression. Dependence and tolerance may also occur.

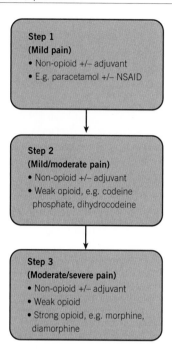

Step 1
(Mild pain)
- Non-opioid +/– adjuvant
- E.g. paracetamol +/– NSAID

Step 2
(Mild/moderate pain)
- Non-opioid +/– adjuvant
- Weak opioid, e.g. codeine phosphate, dihydrocodeine

Step 3
(Moderate/severe pain)
- Non-opioid +/– adjuvant
- Weak opioid
- Strong opioid, e.g. morphine, diamorphine

FIGURE 8.1

Analgesia should be prescribed using the above stepwise regimen. Adjuvant therapies include splints, acupuncture, physiotherapy, occupational therapy and clinical psychology. *(Adapted from the WHO Pain Relief Ladder, available at: http://www.who.int/cancer/palliative/painladder/en/.)*

TABLE 8.1

PARACETAMOL

Uses	Mild to moderate pain Pyrexia
Mechanism of action	Thought to reduce prostaglandin synthesis in CNS Less effective than NSAIDs in controlling inflammatory pain and OA Favoured in the elderly as low risk of GI upset, cardiovascular disease or renal impairment
Side effects	Rash (rare), haematological disorders (rare) Hepatic failure in overdose
Contraindication/caution	No absolute contraindications Caution in hepatic or renal impairment
Recommended dose	0.5–1 g 4–6 hourly, max. 4 g/24 h
Routes of administration	Oral, rectal, intravenous

TABLE 8.2	
OPIOIDS	
Examples	Codeine Dihydrocodeine Tramadol Morphine Oxycodone Fentanyl Targinact (oxycodone and naloxone)*
Uses	Moderate to severe pain
Mechanism of action	Bind to opioid receptors on presynaptic neurones inhibiting pain
Side effects	Nausea and vomiting Constipation, dry mouth Drowsiness and respiratory depression Hypotension Confusion, particularly in the elderly
Contraindication	Respiratory depression. Head injury with reduced conscious level. Ileus
Cautions	Alcohol excess, hepatic or renal impairment Elderly Pregnancy (respiratory depression in neonate), breast-feeding
Recommended dose	Depends on dose and indication. See BNF
Routes of administration	Oral, rectal, intramuscular, intravenous, subcutaneous, transdermal

*Less likely to cause constipation than oxycodone alone.

Opioid toxicity is characterized by:

- Sedation
- Pinpoint pupils
- Slow respiration or cyanosis
- Myoclonic jerks
- Confusion or agitation
- Nightmares or hallucinations.

Opioid-induced nausea and vomiting can be managed by antiemetics such as prochlorperazine, ondansetron or metoclopramide. Opioid-induced constipation can be managed with co-prescription of an aperient such as senna 7.5–15 mg at night. A combination product containing oxycodone and naloxone is also available (Targinact) in which constipation is prevented because naloxone blocks opiate receptors in the gut.

Compound Analgesics

These are fixed dose combinations of paracetamol and a weak opioid such as codeine or dihydrocodeine. They are typically used for moderate pain that is incompletely responsive to paracetamol and where NSAIDs are contraindicated, but they can also be used in combination with NSAIDs. Commonly used preparations include:

TABLE 8.3

NONSTEROIDAL ANTIINFLAMMATORY DRUGS

Examples	Ibuprofen
	Diclofenac
	Naproxen
	Celecoxib (COX-2 selective)
	Etoricoxib (COX-2 selective)
Uses	Inflammatory arthritis (RA, AS, PsA)
	Osteoarthritis
	Bone metastases
	Perioperative pain
	Pyrexia
Mechanism of action	Reduced production of prostaglandins due to inhibition of cyclooxygenase enzymes (Figure 8.2), suppressing inflammation and reducing pain. Nonselective NSAIDs also inhibit COX-1, which is important for protection of the GI mucosa
Side effects	GI upset and peptic ulceration (less likely with COX-2 selective drugs)
	Renal impairment, fluid retention and hypertension
	Increased risk of myocardial infarction and stroke
	Rash, bronchospasm
	May have an inhibitory effect on bone healing
Contraindications	Renal impairment, cardiovascular disease, heart failure, bleeding diathesis, peptic ulcer
Cautions	Asthma, inflammatory bowel disease, pregnancy, breast-feeding, elderly
Recommended dose	Ibuprofen: 200–800 mg t.i.d., max. 2.4 g daily
	Diclofenac: 50 mg t.i.d., max. 150 mg daily
	Celecoxib: 100 mg b.d., max. 400 mg daily
	Naproxen: 500 mg t.i.d, max. 1500 mg daily
	Etoricoxib: 60 mg daily, max. 120 mg
Routes of administration	Ibuprofen: oral, topical
	Diclofenac: oral, rectal, intramuscular, intravenous, topical
	Naproxen: oral
	Celecoxib: oral
	Etoricoxib: oral

- Cocodamol: 8 mg, 15 mg or 30 mg codeine and 500 mg paracetamol. The normal dose is 2 tablets every 6 hours up to a maximum of 8 tablets per day.
- Codydramol: 10 mg, 20 mg or 30 mg dihydrocodeine and 500 mg paracetamol. The normal dose is 2 tablets every 6 hours up to a maximum of 8 tablets per day.

Adverse effects and contraindications/cautions are those described for paracetamol and opioids.

Nonsteroidal Antiinflammatory Drugs

Non-steroidal anti-inflammatory drugs (NSAIDs) inhibit cyclooxygenase (COX) enzymes that are responsible for the production of prostaglandins in

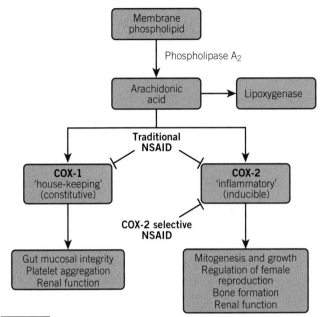

FIGURE 8.2

COX is an enzyme that converts arachidonic acid into prostaglandins. NSAIDs inhibit this action. *(Adapted from Davidson's Principles and Practice of Medicine 22nd Edition (with permission).)*

various tissues. The COX1 enzyme is constitutively expressed in the gastric mucosa, the kidney and platelets. In contrast, COX2 is not constitutively expressed but is upregulated in response to inflammation or injury (Figure 8.2). Nonselective NSAIDs such as ibuprofen and naproxen inhibit both isoforms equally, whereas celecoxib and etoricoxib preferentially inhibit the COX2 enzyme. The COX-2 selective NSAIDs are less likely to cause GI adverse effects than nonselective NSAIDs. All NSAIDs are associated with an increased risk of cardiovascular disease, possibly because of their effects on platelets and tendency to cause fluid retention and raise blood pressure.

- Systemic NSAIDs are effective agents for the treatment of inflammatory pain, osteoarthritis and postoperative pain.
- Topical NSAIDs have a good safety profile and are useful for patients with soft tissue rheumatism and osteoarthritis.
- NSAIDs are contraindicated in patients with cardiovascular disease and heart failure as well as patients with a history of peptic ulcers or GI bleeding.
- NSAIDs should be used with extreme caution in the elderly and in patients with renal impairment.

Because of the risk of GI events with NSAIDs it has been recommended by the UK National Institute for Health and Care Excellence (NICE) that a proton pump inhibitor (e.g. omeprazole) should be co-prescribed with NSAIDs (including COX2 selective NSAIDs). Note that patients with GI ulceration may not have symptoms of dyspepsia. The risk factors for NSAID-induced GI adverse effects include:

- Age >60 years
- Previous history of GI ulceration
- Concomitant corticosteroid treatment.

Antineuropathic Pain Medications

Several medications are available for the treatment of pain associated with damage to or dysfunction of the neural pathways responsible for sensing pain, such as complex regional pain syndromes, fibromyalgia and chronic pain syndrome. They include antiepileptic agents such as gabapentin, selective serotonin reuptake inhibitors (SSRIs) such as fluoxetine, serotonin/ noradrenalin reuptake inhibitors (SNRIs) such as duloxetine and antidepressants such as amitriptyline, which in low doses has SNRI/SSRI properties (Table 8.4).

TABLE 8.4	
ANTI-NEUROPATHIC AGENTS	
Examples	Amitriptyline
	Fluoxetine
	Duloxetine
	Gabapentin
Uses	Neuropathic pain
	Chronic regional pain syndromes
	Fibromyalgia
Mechanism of action	Amytriptyline and duloxetine: inhibit reuptake of serotonin and norepinephrine by presynaptic neurones
	Fluoxetine: inhibits reuptake of serotonin by presynaptic neurones
	Gabapentin: inhibits α_2-δ subunit of voltage-gated calcium channels on postsynaptic neurones
Side effects	Amitriptyline and duloxetine: drowsiness, confusion, dry mouth, urinary retention, weight gain, orthostatic hypotension
	Fluoxetine: nausea, dizziness, dry mouth, sexual dysfunction (selective serotonin re-uptake inhibitors)
	Gabapentin: dizziness, somnolence, oedema, gait disturbance
Contraindications	Amitriptyline: cardiac arrhythmia, recent myocardial infarction, porphyria, hypomania
	Fluoxetine: hypomania
	Duloxetine: myasthenia gravis, bladder outflow obstruction, GI obstruction, bowel hypotonia, severe ulcerative colitis
Cautions	All drugs: elderly, epilepsy, cardiac disease, arrhythmias, diabetes, glaucoma. See BNF for more details

TABLE 8.4	
ANTI-NEUROPATHIC AGENTS—cont'd	
Recommended dose	Amitriptyline: 10–75 mg at night
	Fluoxetine: 20–60 mg daily
	Gabapentin: 300–1200 mg t.i.d
	Duloxetine: 60–120 mg daily
Routes of administration	Amitriptyline: oral
	Fluoxetine: oral
	Duloxetine: oral
	Gabapentin: oral

 HINTS AND TIPS

PAIN MANAGEMENT

The WHO pain ladder is an important tool when determining the appropriate analgesia to prescribe, with the additive effects of analgesia being important. However, the ladder is more suited to the setting of acute rather than chronic pain, where specialist input may be required. When acutely assessing a patient with a decreased conscious level and respiratory rate, always consider opiate toxicity. The short-acting opioid antagonist naloxone can be used to reverse toxicity. Prescription of NSAIDs should be avoided where possible in elderly patients, in the presence of renal or known peptic ulcer disease, or in patients with problems associated with fracture healing.

CORTICOSTEROIDS

Corticosteroids have powerful antiinflammatory and immunosuppressive effects and are widely used in the treatment of inflammatory rheumatic diseases such as SLE, RA, vasculitis and polymyalgia rheumatica. Local steroid injections can be helpful in the treatment of soft tissue disorders (e.g. tennis elbow, golfer's elbow, rotator cuff impingement). Intraarticular steroids have a role in the treatment of inflammatory arthritis and osteoarthritis. Details are provided in Table 8.5.

- High doses of steroids have a key role at inducing remission in GCA, systemic vasculitis, and SLE.
- Low-dose steroids have a role in maintaining remission in vasculitis, SLE and RA. In this situation the dose should be as low as possible to maintain control of the disease.
- Steroid-sparing agents such as azathioprine or methotrexate should be considered in addition to steroids when the maintenance prednisolone dose cannot be reduced below 10 mg daily.
- Long-term corticosteroid use can lead to various complications including diabetes, hypertension and osteoporosis. Prophylaxis against osteoporosis should be considered in these patients (see Drugs for Bone Diseases).

TABLE 8.5

CORTICOSTEROIDS

Examples	Prednisolone Methylprednisolone Hydrocortisone
Uses	Inflammatory arthritis SLE, vasculitis, polymyositis and dermatomyositis Giant cell arteritis (GCA)/poylmyalgia rheumatica (PMR)
Mechanism of action	Multiple, including apoptosis of leukocytes
Side effects	Hypertension, weight gain, fluid retention, easy bruising, thinning of skin, osteoporosis, osteonecrosis, alteration of mood, peptic ulcers, acute pancreatitis, Cushing syndrome, diabetes, myopathy, growth retardation (children)
Contraindication	Active infection
Cautions	Renal, liver or heart failure Peptic ulcers, acute pancreatitis Cushing syndrome, diabetes, hypertension, osteoporosis Avoid live vaccines Pregnancy, breast-feeding (can be used under specialist supervision)
Recommended dose	Dependent on route and indication (see BNF)
Routes of administration	Prednisolone: oral, intramuscular Methylprednisolone: intramuscular, intravenous, intraarticular Hydrocortisone: oral, intramuscular, intravenous Hydrocortisone acetate: intraarticular, soft tissue

---

 HINTS AND TIPS

CORTICOSTEROIDS

Patients on long-term corticosteroids may require an increase in their maintenance dose at the time of concomitant illness or surgery. Always warn patients undergoing a steroid joint injection about the risk of steroid flare, that may result in increased pain for 48 hours.

DISEASE MODIFYING ANTIRHEUMATIC DRUGS

Disease modifying antirheumatic drugs (DMARDs) is the collective name given to a group of small molecule drugs that have immunomodulatory effects. Details of the most commonly used drugs are summarized in Tables 8.6–8.14. Additional DMARDs not discussed here include intramuscular gold (Myocrisin), oral gold (Auranofin), and penicillamine (Distamine). While these drugs are effective in a proportion of patients, adverse effects are common and only a small proportion of patients can be maintained on treatment in the long term. They have been largely superseded by the agents that are discussed in more detail below. Methotrexate is generally considered to be the core DMARD for the treatment of RA, and is often used as the first choice for PsA, and other seronegative inflammatory arthropathies. Apremilast is a small

Text continued on p. 281

TABLE 8.6

METHOTREXATE

Uses	RA
	Seronegative spondyloarthritis
	SLE
	Vasculitis
	GCA/PMR
Mechanism of action	Inhibition of DNA synthesis through dihydrofolate reductase inhibition, thereby causing immunosuppression
Side effects	Mouth ulcers
	Nausea, anorexia
	Alopecia
	Abnormal LFTs, cirrhosis
	Bone marrow suppression
	Hypersensitivity pneumonitis
	Increased risk of infection
Contraindications	Pregnancy* (teratogenic), breast-feeding (discontinue), alcohol excess, infection, immunodeficiency
Cautions	Elderly, hepatic or renal impairment, ascites or pleural effusions
Recommended dose	5–25 mg once weekly
	Folic acid 5 mg weekly the day after methotrexate to reduce side effects
Routes of administration	Oral, subcutaneous

*Contraception is essential during and for 3 months after stopping treatment for both men and women.

TABLE 8.7

AZATHIOPRINE

Uses	SLE and vasculitis
	Giant cell arthritis/PMR
	RA
	Seronegative spondyloarthritis
Mechanism of action	A cytotoxic agent that inhibits DNA synthesis, thereby causing immunosuppression
Adverse effects	Bone marrow suppression
	Abnormal LFTs
	Nausea, vomiting, diarrhoea
	Malaise, dizziness
	Interstitial nephritis
	Increased risk of infection
	Alopecia
Contraindications	Hypersensitivity to azathioprine or mercaptopurine
Cautions	Active infection
	Live vaccines
	Hepatic or renal impairment.
	Pregnancy, breast-feeding (can be used under specialist supervision)
Recommended dose	1–2 mg/kg/day
Route of administration	Oral

TABLE 8.8

CYCLOPHOSPHAMIDE

Uses	SLE Systemic vasculitis
Mechanism of action	An alkylating agent that forms cross-links between strands of DNA, halting cell replication and division, thereby causing immunosuppression
Side effects	Nausea, anorexia, vomiting Bone marrow suppression Cardiac toxicity Alopecia Haemorrhagic cystitis* Increased risk of infection Azoospermia, anovulation
Contraindications	Haemorrhagic cystitis Acute porphyria
Caution	Diabetes, hepatic or renal impairment Pregnancy (teratogenic), breast-feeding (discontinue)
Recommended dose	Oral: 2 mg/kg/day Intravenous: 15 mg/kg every 3–4 weeks on 6–8 occasions
Routes of administration	Oral, intravenous

*Patients receiving cyclophosphamide should be prescribed mesna and be advised to take large volumes of fluid to reduce the risk of this complication.

TABLE 8.9

SULFASALAZINE

Uses	RA Seronegative spondyloarthritis
Mechanism of action	Incompletely understood, but scavenges proinflammatory reactive oxygen species and reduces T-cell activation
Side effects	Nausea, abdominal pain, weight loss Acute pancreatitis, renal or hepatic dysfunction Rash, lupus erythematosus-type syndrome Bone marrow suppression Urine discolouration (orange) Infertility (reversible)
Contraindication	Sulfonamide hypersensitivity
Caution	Renal or hepatic impairment Porphyria Pregnancy, breast-feeding (can be used under specialist supervision)
Recommended dose	500 mg daily, increasing to 3–4 g/day in divided doses
Route of administration	Oral

TABLE 8.10

HYDROXYCHLOROQUINE

Uses	RA SLE
Mechanism of action	Inhibits lysozyme function and antigen processing
Side effects	Retinopathy* with long-term use Nausea, vomiting, diarrhoea, weight loss Rash, headache, skin and hair changes/discolouration Bone marrow suppression
Contraindication	Macular disease
Cautions	Elderly, visual impairment Hepatic or renal impairment Epilepsy, myasthenia gravis, psoriasis, porphyria Alcohol excess Pregnancy (can be used under specialist supervision), breast-feeding (discontinue)
Recommended dose	200–400 mg/day (<6.5 mg/kg)
Route of administration	Oral

*Visual acuity tests should be performed at baseline and ophthalmological advice sought if abnormality detected. The risk of retinopathy increases after 5 years therapy and checks of visual acuity should be performed at 5 years and annually thereafter.

TABLE 8.11

LEFLUNOMIDE

Uses	RA Psoriatic arthritis
Mechanism of action	Specifically inhibits DNA synthesis in lymphocytes, thereby causing immunosuppression
Side effects	Nausea, vomiting, diarrhoea, weight loss Hypertension, headaches, tenosynovitis Alopecia, rash Bone marrow suppression Renal or hepatic dysfunction Increased risk of infection
Contraindications	Infection Immunodeficiency
Cautions	Renal or hepatic disease Pregnancy* (teratogenic), breast-feeding (discontinue)
Recommended dose	10–20 mg/day
Route of administration	Oral

*Contraception is essential during and for 2 years after treatment in women and during and for 3 months after treatment in men.

TABLE 8.12

CICLOSPORIN

Uses	RA
Mechanism of action	Inhibits calcineurin an intracellular signalling molecule involved in activation of T-cells
Side effects	GI upset Malignant or refractory hypertension Renal failure Gingival hyperplasia Electrolyte disturbances Hyperglycaemia, hyperuricaemia
Contraindications	Renal impairment Uncontrolled hypertension
Cautions	Hypertension Hepatic or renal impairment Pregnancy (can be used following careful risk–benefit assessment), breast-feeding (discontinue)
Recommended dose	2.5–4 mg/kg/24 h
Route of administration	Oral

TABLE 8.13

MYCOPHENOLATE MOFETIL

Uses	SLE Vasculitis
Mechanism of action	Inhibits DNA synthesis in lymphocytes
Side effects	GI upset Renal impairment Gingival hyperplasia Electrolyte disturbances Hypogammaglobulinaemia Increased risk of infection Bronchiectasis
Contraindications	Pregnancy* (teratogenic), breast-feeding (discontinue)
Cautions	Elderly, Preexisting GI disease
Recommended dose	2–4 g daily
Route of administration	Oral

*Contraception is essential during and for 6 weeks after treatment in women and men.

TABLE 8.14	
PHOSPHOESTERASE E4 INHIBITORS	
Examples	Apremilast
Uses	PsA
Mechanism of action	Inhibits phosphoesterase D4 in leukocytes which inhibits production of several proinflammatory cytokines, reducing inflammation
Side effects	GI upset Increased risk of infection Weight loss Depression
Contraindications	Hypersensitivity to drug or excipients
Cautions	Pregnancy (no information), breast-feeding (not advised) Renal impairment, history of depression
Recommended dose	30 mg b.d.
Route of administration	Oral

molecule inhibitor of phosphodiesterase E4, which has recently been licensed to treat psoriasis and PsA. The role in treatment remains to be established, but it has been shown to be efficacious in patients that have not responded adequately to standard therapies. Early use of DMARDs with a treat-to-target philosophy aimed at controlling inflammation has been shown to improve clinical outcome in RA:

- Combination DMARDs are frequently used in RA patients that do not respond adequately to a single agent.
- Bone marrow suppression and abnormal LFT are adverse effects of many DMARDs, necessitating blood monitoring for evidence of toxicity, with dose reduction as appropriate.

BIOLOGICAL ANTIRHEUMATIC DRUGS

Biological antirheumatic drugs are used in the treatment of inflammatory rheumatic diseases where the response to combination DMARDs has been inadequate. Details are summarized in Tables 8.15–8.18. The majority of these drugs are monoclonal antibodies directed against specific cytokines or cell surface receptors (Figure 8.3). They have powerful immunomodulatory effects. While often highly effective, treatment is associated with an increased risk of serious infections and of certain malignancies.

 HINTS AND TIPS

DMARDS AND BIOLOGICAL ANTIRHEUMATIC DRUGS

DMARDs and biological antirheumatic drugs play a central role in the medical management of RA and other inflammatory joint diseases, since there is evidence that they favourably alter disease outcome. Biological treatments are usually stopped preoperatively since there is evidence that continued treatment increases the risk of infection. Regular monitoring of full blood count and LFTs are important in patients on many DMARDs, in order to screen for possible adverse effects.

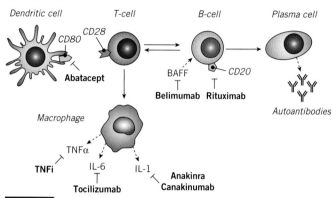

FIGURE 8.3

Biological antirheumatic drugs and their targets. The biological drugs used in the treatment of inflammatory rheumatic diseases target inflammatory cytokines or their receptors (TNFα, IL-6, IL-1), the B-cell growth factor BAFF, the surface marker CD20, or interrupt the CD28-CD80 interaction that is required for T-cell activation.

TABLE 8.15

ANTI-TNF THERAPY

Examples	Infliximab
	Adalimumab
	Certolizumab
	Golimumab
	Etanercept*
Uses	RA
	Psoriatic arthritis
	Ankylosing spondylitis
Mechanism of action	Blocks effects of the proinflammatory cytokine TNFα, thereby reducing inflammation
Side effects	GI upset
	Heart failure
	Increased risk of infection
	Reactivation of TB
	Hypersensitivity reactions
	Injection site reactions
	Increased risk of skin cancer
Contraindications	Active Infection
	Heart failure
	Malignancy
	Demyelinating disease
	Pregnancy (no information),† breast-feeding (discontinue)
Caution	History of infections
Recommended dose	Depends on preparation. See BNF
Routes of administration	Intravenous, subcutaneous

*Etanercept is a decoy receptor for TNFα; the other drugs are monoclonal antibodies to TNFα.

†Contraception is advised during and after treatment with TNFi therapy. Depends on preparation. See BNF for more details.

TABLE 8.16

ANTI-B-CELL THERAPY

Examples	Rituximab Belimumab
Uses	RA (rituximab) ANCA positive vasculitis (rituximab) SLE (Belimumab)
Mechanism of action	Rituximab: monoclonal antibody to CD20, which is expressed on B cells. Binding of rituximab causes complement-mediated destruction of B-cells. Belimumab: blocks effects of B-lymphocyte stimulator, which inhibits B-cell survival and function
Side effects	GI upset Increased risk of infection Infusion reactions Progressive multifocal leukoencephalopathy (rituximab) Leukopenia
Contraindications	Active infection Heart failure Malignancy Pregnancy,* breast-feeding (discontinue)
Caution	History of infections
Recommended dose	Depends on preparation. See BNF
Routes of administration	Intravenous

*Contraception is essential during and after treatment for both men and women.

TABLE 8.17

ANTI-IL-6 THERAPY

Examples	Tocilizumab
Uses	RA
Mechanism of action	Antibody to IL-6 receptor which blocks binding of IL-6 thereby reducing inflammation
Side effects	GI upset Mouth ulcers Increased risk of infection Infusion reactions Abnormal LFT Neutropenia, thrombocytopenia Hypercholesterolemia Diverticulitis
Contraindications	Active infection Pregnancy,* breast-feeding (discontinue)
Caution	History of infections
Recommended dose	8 mg/kg once monthly
Routes of administration	Intravenous, subcutaneous

*Contraception is essential for 3 months before and after treatment in women.

TABLE 8.18

ANTI-IL-1 THERAPY

Examples	Anakinra*
	Canakinumab*
Uses	RA; adult onset Still disease; familial fever syndromes (anakinra)
	Familial fever syndromes; systemic onset juvenile idiopathic
	arthritis, acute gout (canakinumab)
Mechanism of action	Inhibition of IL-1 signalling which reduces inflammation
Side effects	Injection site reactions
	Headache
	Increased risk of infection
	Neutropenia infusion reactions
Contraindications	Neutropenia
	Pregnancy (avoid), breast-feeding (discontinue)
Caution	History of infections; asthma (risk of infection)
Recommended dose	Anakinra: 100 mg daily
	Canakinumab: 150 mg every 8 weeks for adults over 40 kg
Route of administration	Subcutaneous

*Anakinra is an antagonist at the IL-1 receptor, whereas canakinumab is a monoclonal antibody to IL-1β.

DRUGS FOR BONE DISEASES

Drugs for the treatment of bone diseases can be subdivided into those that inhibit osteoclast activity (antiresorptive drugs) and those that stimulate bone formation (anabolic drugs). Calcium and vitamin D supplements are widely used as an adjunct to other treatments for bone disease but may also be used as stand alone treatment in elderly patients who often have a poor diet and are at risk of vitamin D deficiency. Details are summarized in Tables 8.19–8.27.

 HINTS AND TIPS

DRUGS FOR BONE DISEASES

Anti-osteoporosis treatments reduce but do not completely prevent fractures occurring. If a patient fractures on therapy, compliance should be checked and the treatment continued unless there is evidence on BMD testing that the drug is not working. Pathological atypical femoral fractures are a rare complication of long-term therapy with bisphosphonates and other antiresorptive drugs. Hormone replacement therapy is a useful option in younger women with osteoporosis, but adverse effects increase with long-term therapy and those over 60 years.

Text continued on p. 289

TABLE 8.19

BISPHOSPHONATES

Examples	Alendronic acid Risedronate Ibandronate Zoledronic acid Pamidronate
Uses	Osteoporosis Paget disease of bone Metastatic bone disease Cancer-associated hypercalcaemia
Mechanism of action	Inhibition of osteoclastic bone resorption
Side effects	Dyspepsia, heartburn abdominal pain Oesophageal ulceration Bone pain Hypocalcaemia (i.v. use) Renal impairment Atypical femoral fractures Atrial fibrillation (Zoledronic acid) Osteonecrosis of the jaw (dose related)
Contraindications	Dysphagia, oesophageal stricture, achalasia Renal impairment, hypocalcaemia
Cautions	Barrett oesophagus Recent GI ulceration or bleeding Pregnancy (avoid while on treatment), breast-feeding (no information)
Recommended dose	Depends on drug and indication. See BNF
Routes of administration	Oral (fasting): wait at least 30 min before taking food or other medications; intravenous

TABLE 8.20

RANKL INHIBITORS

Examples	Denosumab
Uses	Osteoporosis Metastatic bone disease
Mechanism of action	Monoclonal antibody which blocks effect of RANKL, inhibiting osteoclastic bone resorption
Side effects	Hypocalcaemia Atypical femoral fractures Osteonecrosis of the jaw Erysipelas
Contraindications	Hypocalcaemia
Cautions	Pregnancy (avoid while o treatment) breast feeding (no information)
Recommended dose	Osteoporosis: 60 mg every 6 months Metastatic bone disease: 120 mg every month
Route of administration	Subcutaneous injection

TABLE 8.21

PARATHYROID HORMONE

Examples	Teriparatide
Uses	Osteoporosis
Mechanism of action	Stimulation of bone turnover which stimulates bone formation more than bone resorption, increasing bone mass
Side effects	Muscle cramps, headache GI upset, dizziness, breathlessness Hypercalcaemia (treatment can usually be continued)
Contraindications	Skeletal malignancy Previous radiotherapy to bone Paget disease Hypercalcaemia Renal impairment Unexplained elevation in alkaline phosphatase
Cautions	Pregnancy (avoid), breast-feeding (avoid)
Recommended dose	20 µg/day for 2 years
Route of administration	Subcutaneous

TABLE 8.22

STRONTIUM RANELATE

Uses	Osteoporosis
Mechanism of action	Incompletely understood. Inhibits bone turnover and also substitutes for calcium in hydroxyapatite
Side effects	Upper GI upset and diarrhoea Headache Skin rashes Allergic reactions Increased risk of VTE Increased risk of cardiovascular disease
Contraindications	Cardiovascular disease Renal impairment
Caution	History of VTE
Recommended dose	2 g daily
Route of administration	Oral (fasting, wait 2 hours before taking food)

TABLE 8.23

HORMONE REPLACEMENT THERAPY

Examples	Prempak C (conjugated oestrogen and norgesterel) Kliovance (oestradiol and norethisterone) Estraderm MR (oestradiol)
Uses	Osteoporosis, treatment of menopausal symptoms
Mechanism of action	Suppresses bone turnover resulting from oestrogen deficiency
Side effects	Fluid retention, weight gain, headaches, menstrual bleeding Increased risk of venous thromboembolism Increased risk of breast and endometrial cancer with long-term use Increased risk of stroke, cardiovascular disease with long-term use
Contraindications	Hormone dependent cancer, previous VTE
Cautions	Migraine Risk factors for VTE Liver disease Pregnancy, breast-feeding
Recommended dose	Depends on drug. See BNF
Routes of administration	Oral, transdermal

TABLE 8.24

SELECTIVE OESTROGEN RECEPTOR MODULATORS

Examples	Raloxifene Tibolone
Uses	Osteoporosis Vasomotor symptoms (tibolone)
Mechanism of action	Raloxifene: selective oestrogen receptor modulator which acts as an oestrogen receptor agonist in bone and endometrium but an antagonist in breast and vascular tissues Tibolone: partial agonist of oestrogen, androgen and progesterone receptors
Side effects	Raloxifene: hot flushes, leg cramps, fluid retention, increased risk of VTE Tibolone: GI upset, menstrual bleeding, hirsutism, weight gain, fluid retention
Contraindications	Venous thromboembolism, endometrial cancer (raloxifene) Cerebrovascular disease (tibolone)
Cautions	Breast cancer,* endometrial cancer Risk factors for VTE (raloxifene) Liver disease, renal disease Pregnancy (not advised), breast-feeding (discontinue)
Recommended dose	Raloxifene: 60 mg/day Tibolone: 2.5 mg daily
Route of administration	Oral

*Although this is listed as a caution, data from clinical trials show that long-term use of raloxifene is associated with a significantly reduced risk of breast cancer.

TABLE 8.25

CALCITONIN

Uses	Paget disease
	Hypercalcaemia
Mechanism of action	Osteoclast inhibitor
Side effects	GI upset,
	Flushes, headache, dizziness
	Hypersensitivity reactions
	Increased risk of malignancy
Contraindication	Hypocalcaemia
Cautions	Hypersensitivity
	Renal impairment
	Cardiac failure
	Pregnancy (avoid), breast-feeding (discontinue)
Recommended dose	100 units t.i.d. (hypercalcaemia)
	50 units 3 times weekly to 100 units daily (Paget's)
Route of administration	Subcutaneous

TABLE 8.26

CALCIUM AND VITAMIN D

Examples	Adcal D3 (cholecalciferol and calcium)
	Calcichew D3 (cholecalciferol and calcium)
	Calfovit D3 (colecalciferol and calcium)
Uses	Dietary calcium and vitamin D deficiency
	Vitamin D deficiency
	Osteomalacia
Mechanism of action	Correct dietary deficiency
	Correction of secondary hyperparathyroidism
Side effects	GI upset
	Constipation
Contraindication	Hypercalcaemia
Caution	Renal stone disease
Recommended dose	Adcal D3 and Calcichew D3: 1–2 daily
	Calfovit D3: 1–2 sachets daily
Route of administration	Oral

TABLE 8.27

VITAMIN D

Examples	Fultium D3 (cholecalciferol)
	InvitaD3 (cholecalciferol)
	Alfacalcidol (calcidiol)
	Rocaltrol (calcitriol)
Uses	Vitamin D deficiency
	Osteomalacia
	Renal osteodystrophy, hypoparathyroidism (alfacalcidol, rocaltrol)
Mechanism of action	Increases intestinal calcium absorption
Side effects	Hypercalcaemia
Contraindications	Hypercalcaemia
Cautions	Renal stone disease, sarcoidosis
Recommended dose	Fultium D3: 800–1600 units daily
	InvitaD3: 25,000 units once a month
	Alfacalcidol: 0.5–4 mcg daily
	Rocaltrol: 0.25–2 mcg daily
Route of administration	Oral

HYPERURICAEMIA AND GOUT

Drugs for the treatment of gout can be subdivided into those used to treat an acute attack and those used to control hyperuricaemia to prevent attacks occurring. Details are provided in Tables 8.28–8.30.

Treatment of the acute attack:

- First line: colchicine 500 μg 2–3 times daily or oral NSAIDs
- Second line: oral prednisolone 15–20 mg daily for 3–5 days or intraarticular methylprednisolone
- A high-fluid intake should be encouraged.

Long-term control of hyperuricaemia:

- Allopurinol 100 mg daily, increasing gradually to 900 mg daily until serum urate <360 μmol/L
- Febuxostat 60 mg daily increasing to 120 mg daily to reduce and maintain serum urate <360 μmol/L
- Colchicine or NSAIDs cover is usually given during first 6 months of urate lowering therapy to reduce the risk of acute attacks
- Reduce alcohol intake, weight loss and avoid purine rich foods.

 HINTS AND TIPS

HYPERURICAEMIA AND GOUT

There is an increased risk of acute gout attacks when initiating urate lowering therapy. The risk of this can be reduced by slowly increasing the dose of allopurinol and the use of prophylactic colchicine or NSAIDs. Urate lowering therapy should not be stopped if acute gout occurs. Treatment should be continued and the acute attack treated.

TABLE 8.28

COLCHICINE

Uses	Acute gout
	Acute pseudogout (unlicensed)
	Familial Mediterranean fever (unlicensed)
	Behçet syndrome (unlicensed)
Mechanism of action	Inhibits microtubule formation in leukocytes which in turn suppressed activation of inflammatory pathways
Side effects	Nausea, vomiting, diarrhoea
	GI bleeding
	Bone marrow suppression
	Renal or hepatic dysfunction
Contraindication	Blood disorders
Cautions	Elderly
	Renal, hepatic or cardiac impairment
	Pregnancy (avoid), breast-feeding (not recommended)
Recommended dose	500 µg 2–3 times daily for 3–4 days in acute gout and pseudogout
	Long-term therapy is required for Behçet syndrome and familial Mediterranean fever
Route of administration	Oral

TABLE 8.29

ALLOPURINOL

Uses	Treatment of hyperuricaemia in patients with gout
Mechanism of action	Inhibits xanthine oxidase, thereby decreasing the production of uric acid
Side effects	Acute gout
	Rash, hypersensitivity
	GI upset
	Headache, hypertension
	Hepatic impairment with the potential for toxicity
	Bone marrow suppression
Contraindication	None
Cautions	Acute gout
	Renal or hepatic impairment
	Pregnancy (use only if necessary), breast-feeding (caution)
Recommended dose	100–900 mg/day
Route of administration	Oral

TABLE 8.30

FEBUXOSTAT

Uses	Treatment of hyperuricaemia in patients with gout
Mechanism of action	Inhibits xanthine oxidase, thereby decreasing the production of uric acid
Side effects	Acute gout Rash GI upset Abnormal LFT Headache Oedema
Contraindication	None
Cautions	Acute gout Renal or hepatic impairment Cardiovascular disease Pregnancy (use only if necessary), breast-feeding (discontinue)
Recommended dose	60–120 mg/day
Route of administration	Oral

ANTICOAGULANTS

The most common anticoagulants encountered within orthopaedics and rheumatology are aspirin, warfarin, heparin and novel oral anticoagulants (NOAC) that act as competitive inhibitors of activated factor X. The details of these drugs are found in Tables 8.31–8.34.

Anticoagulants need to be reviewed and adjusted perioperatively in patients who take them for unrelated disorders, e.g. atrial fibrillation. The need for anticoagulants should be reviewed and the dose may need to be adjusted perioperatively in patients who are taking them for prophylaxis of thromboembolic disorders. They are also used for both the prophylaxis and

TABLE 8.31

ASPIRIN

Uses	Secondary prevention of cardiovascular disease Prophylaxis of DVT and venous thromboembolism (VTE) Pyrexia Pain
Mechanism of action	Irreversible inactivation of COX enzyme (predominantly COX-1), inhibiting production of thromboxane and prostaglandin, stopping platelet aggregation
Side effects	GI upset, peptic ulceration and bleeding Bronchospasm
Contraindications	Hypersensitivity to aspirin/NSAIDs Cerebral bleed Active PUD Bleeding disorders Breast-feeding

Continued

TABLE 8.31

ASPIRIN—cont'd

Cautions	Elderly
	Asthma
	Uncontrolled hypertension
	Hepatic impairment
	Renal impairment
	Pregnancy
	Drug interactions
	G6PD deficiency
	Other anticoagulants
Recommended dose	75 mg once daily
	150 mg once daily (for VTE prophylaxis)
Route of administration	Oral

TABLE 8.32

WARFARIN

Uses	Atrial fibrillation (prevention of stroke)
	Prophylaxis and treatment of DVT and VTE
	Prosthetic heart valves
	Antiphospholipid syndrome (prophylaxis of thrombosis)
Mechanism of action	Inhibits vitamin K 2,3-epoxide reductase and thus vitamin K production within the liver, limiting the production of clotting factors
Side effects	Bleeding
	GI upset
	Jaundice and hepatic dysfunction
	Pancreatitis
	Alopecia
	Purpura/rash
Contraindications	Pregnancy
	Haemorrhagic stroke
	Active peptic ulcer disease
	Active bleeding
Cautions	History of bleeding disorder
	Hepatic impairment
	Renal impairment
	Breast-feeding
	Elderly and high risk of falls
	Drug interactions
	Other anticoagulants
Recommended dose	Loading dose on initiation of treatment
	Maintenance dose guided by INR
	Target INR dependent on indication
Route of administration	Oral

TABLE 8.33

HEPARIN

Examples	Dalteparin (LMWH) Enoxaparin (LMWH) Heparin sodium (unfractionated)*
Uses	Prophylaxis and treatment of DVT and VTE Myocardial infarction Cardiopulmonary bypass surgery Haemodialysis Perioperative anticoagulation in patients at high risk of bleeding
Mechanism of action	Binds to antithrombin III inhibiting predominantly thrombin factor Xa
Side effects	Bleeding GI upset Heparin-induced thrombocytopenia Hyperaemia Osteoporosis (low risk with LMWH) Alopecia Injection site irritation
Contraindications	Thrombocytopenia including heparin-induced thrombocytopenia Cerebral bleed Uncontrolled hypertension Active PUD Bleeding disorders including active bleeding Hypersensitivity Significant risk of major bleeding
Cautions	History of bleeding disorder Hepatic impairment Renal impairment Elderly Drug interactions Other anticoagulants
Recommended dose	Depends on form and indication. See BNF
Routes of administration	Intravenous, subcutaneous

*Requires regular monitoring using APTT.

TABLE 8.34

NOVEL ORAL ANTICOAGULANTS

Examples	Rivaroxaban Apixaban
Uses	Prophylaxis and treatment of VTE Atrial fibrillation
Mechanism of action	Binds to activated factor X (factor Xa), which it directly inhibits
Side effects	Bleeding GI upset Hypotension Dizziness and headache Renal impairment Pruritus or rash Angioedema or jaundice (rare)

Continued

TABLE 8.34

NOVEL ORAL ANTICOAGULANTS—cont'd

Contraindications	Pregnancy
	Breast-feeding
	Liver disease with coagulopathy
	Bleeding disorders including active bleeding
	Significant risk of major bleeding
Cautions	History of bleeding disorder
	Hepatic impairment
	Renal impairment
	Severe hypertension
	Vascular retinopathy
	Elderly and high risk of falls
	Other anticoagulants
	Anaesthesia with postop indwelling epidural catheter
	Bronchiectasis
Recommended dose	Depends on form and indication. Consult appropriate drug formulary
Route of administration	Oral

management of venous thromboembolism. The therapeutic international normalised ratio (INR) range for warfarin is determined by the indication. Low molecular weight heparin (LMWH) is generally preferred in day-to-day practice, but unfractionated heparin is used in those at high risk of bleeding as the anticoagulant effect can be stopped by stopping the infusion. Several novel oral anticoagulants have been found to be effective in the prevention of postoperative deep venous thrombosis (DVT) and they have the advantage that they do not require monitoring.

 HINTS AND TIPS

ANTICOAGULANTS

For patients due to undergo elective surgery, warfarin is usually discontinued approximately 5 days prior to the proposed procedure. Vitamin K may be required in the acute setting with a trauma patient. Heparin (LMWH or unfractionated if required) can be used in the perioperative period to bridge until warfarin is recommenced and within the therapeutic range. LMWH should not increase the activated partial thromboplastin time (APTT), but unfractionated heparin will. The patient should be recommenced on warfarin postoperatively, the timing of which is dependent on the surgery and postoperative course but can usually be done within the first 48 hours. Bridging heparin is routinely continued until the INR is within the therapeutic range.

Bibliography and Further Reading

Adebajo A. ABC of Rheumatology. 3rd ed. Wiley–Blackwell: BMJ Books; 2009.

American College of Surgeons Committee on Trauma. ATLS Student Manual. 9th ed. Chicago: American College of Surgeons; 2012.

Ballinger A, Patchett S. Essentials of Kumar and Clark's Clinical Medicine. 5th ed. Saunders; 2011.

British National Formulary: Current Edition

Chalmers C, Parchment-Smith C. MRCS Part A: Essential Revision Notes Book 1 and Book 2. 1st ed. PasTest; 2012.

Chatu S. The Hands-on Guide to Clinical Pharmacology. 3rd ed. Wiley–Blackwell; 2010.

Collier J, Longmore M, Amarakone K. Oxford Handbook of Clinical Specialties. 9th ed. Oxford: Oxford University Press; 2013.

Dandy DJ, Edwards DJ. Essential Orthopaedics and Trauma. 5th ed. Elsevier: Churchill Livingstone; 2009.

Davey P. Medicine at a Glance. 4th ed. Wiley–Blackwell; 2014.

Douglas G, Nicol F, Robertson C. MacLeod's Clinical Examination. 13th ed. Elsevier: Churchill Livingstone; 2013.

Drake R, Vogl W, Mitchell A. Gray's Anatomy for Students. 3rd ed. Elsevier: Churchill Livingstone; 2014.

Elias-Jones C, Perry M. Crash Course: Rheumatology and Orthopaedics. 3rd ed. Elsevier: Mosby; 2015.

Ford MJ, Hennessay I, Japp A. Introduction to Clinical Examination. 8th ed. Elsevier: Churchill Livingstone; 2005.

Fuller G, Manford M. Neurology: An Illustrated Colour Text. 3rd ed. Elsevier: Churchill Livingstone; 2010.

Gosling JA, Harris PF, Humpherson JR, Whitmore I, Willan PLT. Human Anatomy: Color Atlas and Textbook. 5th ed. Elsevier: Mosby; 2008.

Gunn C. Bones and Joints: A Guide for Students. 6th ed. Elsevier: Churchill Livingstone; 2012.

Kumar P, Clark ML. Clinical Medicine. 8th ed. Elsevier: Saunders; 2012.

Luqmani RA, Robb J, Porter DE, Joseph B. Textbook of Orthopaedics, Trauma and Rheumatology. 2nd ed. Elsevier: Churchill Livingstone; 2013.

McLatchie GR, Borley N, Chikwe J. Oxford Handbook of Clinical Surgery. 4th ed. Oxford: Oxford University Press; 2013.

McRae R. Clinical Orthopaedic Examination. 6th ed. Elsevier: Churchill Livingstone; 2010.

Moore KL, Agur AMR, Dalley AF. Essential Clinical Anatomy. Lippincott Williams & Wilkins; 2014.

O'Brien M. Aids to the Examination of the Peripheral Nervous System. 5th ed. Edinburgh: Saunders; 2010.

Page CP, Hoffman B, Curtis MJ, Walker MJA. Integrated Pharmacology. 3rd ed. Elsevier: Mosby; 2006.

Panayi GS, Dickson DJ. Churchill's in Clinical Practice Series: Arthritis. 1st ed. Elsevier: Churchill Livingstone; 2004.

Raftery AT, Delbridge MS, Wagstaff MJD. Churchill's Pocketbook of Surgery. 4th ed. Elsevier: Churchill Livingstone; 2011.

Raftery AT, Delbridge MS, Douglas HE. Basic Science for the MRCS. 2nd ed. Elsevier: Churchill Livingstone; 2012.

SIGN Guideline 110: Early management of patients with a head injury. Edinburgh: Health Improvement Scotland; 2009.

SIGN Guideline 111: Management of hip fracture in older people. Edinburgh: Health Improvement Scotland; 2009.

SIGN Guideline 121: Diagnosis and management of psoriasis and psoriatic arthritis in adults. Edinburgh: Quality Improvement Scotland; 2010.

SIGN Guideline 123: Management of early rheumatoid arthritis. Edinburgh: Quality Improvement Scotland; 2011.

SIGN Guideline 142: Management of osteoporosis and the prevention of fragility fractures. Edinburgh: Health Improvement Scotland; 2015.

Solomon L, Warwick DJ, Nayagam S. Apley and Solomon's Concise System of Orthopaedics and Trauma. 4th ed. CRC Press; 2014.

Stenhouse L. Crash Course: Anatomy. 4th ed. Elsevier: Mosby; 2015.

Tornetta P, Court-Brown CM, Heckman JD, McKee M, McQueen MM, Ricci WM. Rockwood and Green's Fractures in Adults. 8th ed. Lippincott Williams & Wilkins; 2014.

Walker BR, Colledge NR, Ralston SH, Penman I. Davidson's Principles and Practice of Medicine. 22nd ed. Elsevier: Churchill Livingstone; 2014.

Watts RA, Conaghan PG, Denton C, Foster H, Issacs J, Müller-Ladner U. Oxford Textbook of Rheumatology. 4th ed. Oxford: Oxford University Press; 2013.

White TO, MacKenzie SP, Gray AJ. McRae's Orthopaedic Trauma and Emergency Fracture Management. 3rd ed. Elsevier: Churchill Livingstone; 2015.

Useful Websites

http://www.bnf.org: Online British National Formulary.

http://www.boa.ac.uk: British Orthopaedic Association.

http://www.nice.org.uk: National Institute for Health and Care Excellence (NICE) management guidelines.

http://www.rheumatology.org.uk: British Society of Rheumatology.

http://www.sign.ac.uk: Scottish Intercollegiate Guidelines Network (SIGN) management guidelines.

Index

Page numbers followed by "*f*" indicate figures, "*b*" indicate boxes, and "*t*" indicate tables.